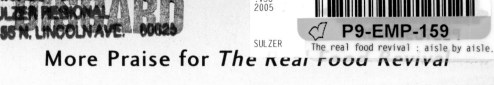

More Praise for *The Real Food Revival*

"*The Real Food Revival* tells you what is wrong with our food—why it is less delightful than it should be. It also tells you what you can do about it—and supplies the two essential, all-too-rare ingredients: truth and hope."

—Margaret Visser, author of *Much Depends on Dinner*

"As someone who heads to the supermarket with both guilt and trepidation, I greeted *The Real Food Revival* as a godsend. It's a passionate and lucidly written guide for the socially conscious eaters among us."

—Steve Almond, author of *Candy Freak*

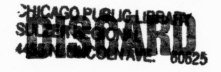

Sherri Brooks Vinton

and

Ann Clark Espuelas

Jeremy P. Tarcher/Penguin

a member of Penguin Group (USA) Inc.

New York

THE
REAL FOOD
REVIVAL

AISLE BY AISLE,
MORSEL BY MORSEL

JEREMY P. TARCHER/PENGUIN
Published by the Penguin Group

Penguin Group (USA) Inc., 375 Hudson Street, New York, New York 10014, USA •
Penguin Group (Canada), 10 Alcorn Avenue, Toronto, Ontario M4V 3B2, Canada
(a division of Pearson Penguin Canada Inc.) • Penguin Books Ltd, 80 Strand, London
WC2R 0RL, England • Penguin Ireland, 25 St Stephen's Green, Dublin 2, Ireland
(a division of Penguin Books Ltd) • Penguin Group (Australia), 250 Camberwell Road,
Camberwell, Victoria 3124, Australia (a division of Pearson Australia Group Pty Ltd) •
Penguin Books India Pvt Ltd, 11 Community Centre, Panchsheel Park, New Delhi–
110 017, India • Penguin Group (NZ), Cnr Airborne and Rosedale Roads, Albany,
Auckland 1310, New Zealand (a division of Pearson New Zealand Ltd.) • Penguin Books
(South Africa) (Pty) Ltd, 24 Sturdee Avenue, Rosebank, Johannesburg 2196, South Africa

Penguin Books Ltd, Registered Offices:
80 Strand, London WC2R 0RL, England

Library of Congress Cataloging-in-Publication Data

Vinton, Sherri Brooks, date.
The real food revival : aisle by aisle, morsel by morsel/
Sherri Brooks Vinton and Ann Clark Espuelas.
p.   cm.
Includes bibliographical references.
ISBN 1-58542-421-8 (alk. paper)
1. Natural foods. 2. Cookery (Natural foods). I. Espuelas, Ann Clark.   II. Title.
TX369.V56   2005   2004065929
641.3'02—dc22

Printed in the United States of America
1   3   5   7   9   10   8   6   4   2

Book design by Meighan Cavanaugh

Most Tarcher/Penguin books are available at special quantity discounts for bulk purchase for
sales promotions, premiums, fund-raising, and educational needs. Special books or book ex-
cerpts also can be created to fit specific needs. For details, write Penguin Group (USA) Inc.
Special Markets, 375 Hudson Street, New York, NY 10014.

While the author has made every effort to provide accurate telephone numbers and Internet addresses at the time of publication, neither the publisher nor the author assumes any responsibility for errors, or for changes that occur after publication. Further, the publisher does
not have any control over and does not assume responsibility for another or third-party Web
sites or their content.

The recipes contained in this book are to be followed exactly as written. The publisher is
not responsible for your specific health or allergy needs that may require supervision. The
publisher is not responsible for any adverse reactions to the recipes contained in this book.

For all the growers and producers working for
a delicious, sustainable future

SBV

For Jack

ACE

CONTENTS

PREFACE

"So, what do you know about food?" Often it was the first question asked when we would tell someone we were working on a book about the topic. The answer is not a lot, at least not in the formal sense. We are not scientists or scholars, chefs or farmers—we certainly are not dieticians. We are eaters. Okay, the kind of voraciously passionate eaters who think Julia Child should be canonized and whose pulses quicken at the sight of spring's first asparagus. More than anything, we are curious eaters.

And that is enough. Because Real Food isn't rocket science; it's common sense. When Sherri was on a cross-country motorcycle trek a few years ago, it didn't take an expert to tell her that something was terribly wrong with our nation's food system. Miles spent with nothing but a helmet to separate her from the crop dusters flying overhead gave her a unique perspective on the use of agricultural chemicals. Months of eating on the road proved that local delicacies—Southern grits and pit beef, New

England clam chowder—were being replaced by the fry-o-lator fare of national fast food chains. Riding through family farming communities turned to ghost towns brought her face-to-face with the specter of corporate ownership that dominates our food supply. When Ann's son was born, she didn't need a survey to suggest that the aisles of "kid-friendly" foods in the grocery store might not be so friendly after all. And that MegaMarts the size of football fields stocked end-to-end with identical displays of processed foods, out-of-season produce, and anonymous meat cuts were crowding out suitable alternatives.

We both had defining moments that led to this project. And we pitched in with different tasks to accomplish it—Sherri, the "I" you hear in the text, did the majority of the writing, Ann the editing.

In our research we found that it doesn't take any special credentials to find Real Food. It just takes eaters who aren't afraid to ask questions. That's what we did and it's all you have to do to reclaim the pleasures of the table—to take charge of where your food comes from, how it was raised, and how it gets to you. In the pages ahead and through the resources provided we hope you will find many of the answers you need to enjoy Real Food. And we hope that you will begin to ask questions of your own, because when you do, you *are* the Real Food Revival.

—Sherri Brooks Vinton
and Ann Clark Espuelas,
June 2005

INTRODUCTION

What Is Real Food?

Peaches. The word even sounds juicy. And that flirt of pink across the vel-
vety cheek of the fruit signals summer flavor. The image is a powerful
childhood memory to me. My Granny Toni was a woman who grew,
canned, dried, pickled, and put-up everything, including peaches, herself.
The peach tree in her yard was, in my mind, the "strudel tree," because
every year when the peaches were ripe for picking we would collect the
fruit (bugs, worms, and all), and, after a good cleaning, she would turn
them into the kind of pastry that dreams are made of. Sweet, sticky, warm,
and buttery—and loaded with the golden jewels that, just a day before,
were hanging on the tree.

Now that's flavor. And it's an ideal that I still seek. But the bushels in
the MegaMart, as plentiful as they are, fail to deliver. I started to wonder,

is it me? Am I just romanticizing about a still-warm-from-the-sun, juice-dripping-down-my-elbow, imperfectly shaped, pristinely flavored peach that perhaps never was? But then I hear more eaters complaining about how food just doesn't taste the same anymore—that you can't get a sweet strawberry these days. Or even worse, I think about the food pleasures that have fallen away unlamented, such as succulent pork chops from carefully raised pigs or the bright saffron yellow of a farm-fresh egg. And I see headlines about food-borne illnesses on the rise, read about trade wars being waged over countries trying to protect their food supply from the controlling hands of agribusiness. And I start to think, can these things be connected? And when did this happen?

Well, the "when" was about 1945. Just after World War II, the food industry in America went through a sea change. Postwar America saw tremendous growth in many areas of development, including agricultural technology. Now, more than fifty years later, advancements designed to help farmers have mutated into industrial agriculture, a heavily consolidated system—controlled by just a handful of corporate agribusinesses—that separates the farmer from the land and relies on chemical and genetic science for its continued survival. This system has a laundry list of negative consequences. Family farms are disappearing and, with them, the small towns that were the backbone of our rural landscape and economy. Agricultural toxins tinge our air, water, soil, even our bloodstreams. And industrial agriculture's centralized growing and distribution model—in producing food designed to travel thousands of miles as it passes through a gauntlet of warehouses and storage facilities—actually robs us of fresh and flavorful things to eat.

For me, it was this matter of taste that drew me into caring about the state of the food chain in the United States. I don't want to live in a world of flavorless, mealy peaches, or any foods, for that matter, that are the product of so-called advances of industrial agriculture—pumped up on grow-fast chemical potions and built for travel.

Isn't that what you want? Food with lots of flavor, maybe even tradition behind its production, but no hidden surprises—no added chemicals to make it grow at record speeds, give it a shelf life longer than table salt, or make it taste "more natural"? And wouldn't it be terrific if you knew that each morsel made it to the end of your fork without scarring the Earth or forcing a farmer into bankruptcy? And perhaps came with a guarantee that future generations would have at least the same—if not better— access to all of the delicious rewards of the table? If you do, you aren't dreaming—and you don't need your own peach tree—you just want what I call "Real Food."

So what do I mean by Real Food? Well, here's what it's not: It's not a trend or a fad. Although you might find some signs that help point the way, Real Food can't be summed up in a label, sticker, or seal. It's not something that you can rely on government agencies, such as the Environmental Protection Agency (EPA), Food and Drug Administration (FDA), or United States Department of Agriculture (USDA), to deliver or even define—charged with protecting the environment, our food supply, and our health, the parameters of these agencies' jurisdictions are often hazy and their standards sometimes in direct conflict. Real Food is not a marketing campaign dreamed up on Madison Avenue and plastered on the side of a bus. In fact, Real Food is nothing new at all. Real Food has been around since man began eating.

It's only in our recent history that defining Real Food—and finding it—has become a challenge. Is it organic? Is it slow? Is it local? Is it sustainable? Is it produced under Fair Trade standards? The answer to all of these questions is yes. And, above all, Real Food is real good. It's one of the great pleasures of life. It shouldn't be a source of anxiety and frustration or a confusing puzzle to untangle—it should be a delight.

So let's start there. What is Real Food? At its most basic, Real Food is:

- Delicious
- Produced as locally as possible
- Sustainable
- Affordable
- Accessible

First of all, Real Food has real flavor. It is produced by people with a genuine interest in what they are doing and the products they are creating. In such operations—whether at the farm, on the boat, at the bakery's ovens, the mill, or the olive press—the taste of the food's the thing, not the happiness of the corporate office, the rewards to shareholders, or the approval of board members.

The second key to the pleasure of Real Food is that it reflects the region in which it was grown. A short distance from field to fork makes for a fresh and tasty meal. Every mile subtracts fragile flavor and adds costs—economic and environmental—to your dish. This means no corn in January if you live in Vermont, but blueberries every which way you can imagine in August.

Real Food is also "sustainable," a word used in many disciplines, from economics to agriculture, to describe an enduring, positive vision for the future of our planet. In terms of food, sustainability connotes several things, all of which imply a keen eye to the long-term impact of its production. As you will see in the chapters ahead, sustainably cultivated fruits, vegetables, and grains are grown with as few chemical inputs as possible, meat is ranched with a sensitivity to animal welfare, and fish are harvested with a respect and understanding of the impact on the oceans. Natural resources such as fresh air and clean water are protected, and biodiversity—the complex distinctiveness of all living things—is preserved.

Real Food is not expensive. If you are smart about your purchases, eating Real Food can actually stretch your grocery dollars further than loading up on conventional items. And as discussed throughout the book, when all factors are taken into account, it is actually "cheap" food that has a higher cost. Eaters pay for such food in farmer subsidies that come out of our taxes; in flavor, which isn't a priority in such goods; and in the damage inflicted on the environment and human health by employing unsavory farming and production techniques to cut corners in the growing process. Real Food exacts none of these costs.

And last, Real Food is accessible—you don't need to live by a farm or near a gourmet store in a big city to find it. And it doesn't require fancy recipes to taste good. You can find it pretty much wherever you shop, and after you read this book you will know how to spot it.

The Revival

So Real Food is delicious, is produced as locally as possible, and is sustainable, affordable, and accessible. Finding and enjoying such food has produced nothing short of a movement— the Real Food Revival. And its followers have all discovered that there's never been a better time to eat in America.

You, the eater—not the dieticians, the advertisers, or the producers— are the most important element of this movement. The eaters drive the market. Each day, most everyone makes choices about food. We cast our votes through vending machines and take-out windows, at the grocery register, and on our restaurant checks. And each vote makes a difference. Every time you choose flavor—for the locally grown apple over the imported one, for the meal at the diner down the block instead of at the drive-thru chain—you are playing a part in the Real Food Revival. And you're not alone.

Farmers inspired by the Real Food Revival are coming to the fields with their minds in the clouds and their hands in the dirt, envisioning a new agrarian future—one that feeds communities without bankrupting natural resources. Through the efforts of devoted growers, produce varieties and livestock breeds on the brink of extinction are making their way back to our plates. Artisanal food producers are rising in number, creating previously hard-to-find, unique products—from sensuous cheeses to luscious chocolate to rustic breads.

Chefs, many inspired by chef and advocate Alice Waters's dedication to Real Food, are building direct relationships with their producers—working around harvest schedules, requesting specific crops, attending tastings, even brainstorming field-plotting plans for the coming year. Maury Rubin of City Bakery in New York City calls his relationships with growers "going to the well," a return to the source of quality and flavor that informs his craft and rewards eaters who seek out treasures such as his signature seasonal tarts.

Equally important is that eaters' demand for quality items is changing the way many retail outlets work. It isn't uncommon to see a designated area for organically grown items in the produce aisles these days. Eaters' requests for local products are also causing food stores to break out of the centralized distribution system that previously shut out small growers. Such venues are working more closely with growers to bring customers food that is fresh from the farm. Throughout the pages ahead, you will read about a number of ways to find Real Food in the aisles of every MegaMart and how to take advantage of additional supply routes outside its doors.

How to Use This Book

This book will not ask you to change what you like to eat. It will not ask you to become a vegetarian. It will not ask you to abstain from fat, adopt a high-protein, low-anything diet. This is a book of celebration and indulgence, an ode to culinary delight. It provides a real-world guide to hunting out the best food there is to be had and a note of gratitude for epicurean diversity. And in the chapters ahead, you'll find all the tools you need to join in this feast.

Each *Aisle* is devoted to a specific food group and gives you the why, where, and how of eating Real Food. The Aisles are broken down into several sections. The *Industrial Agriculture Snapshot* gives you a glimpse of the state of food production in terms of each particular food group—pointing out the impact of these methods on the environment, the economy, the community, and ourselves. *Reviving Real Food* gives you actions big and small that you can take—wherever you shop—to bring home the best food available. The remaining chapter gives you information about some grocery stores that are working to make your search for sustainably produced food easier, as well as a directory of print and online sources for eaters who want to become more involved in the Real Food Revival.

So pick up a fork and turn the page. It's time for some Real Food.

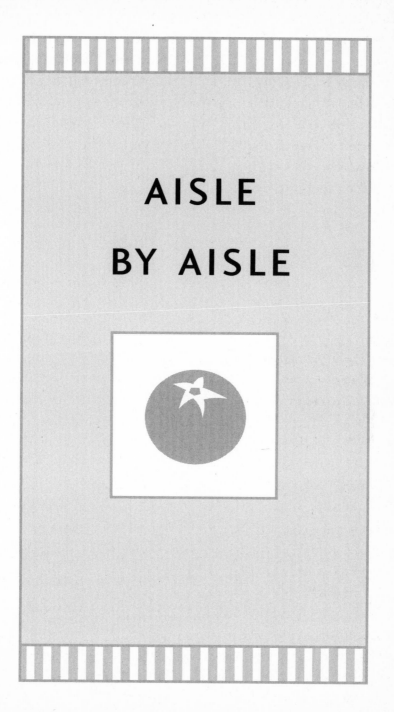

AISLE
BY AISLE

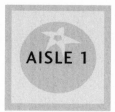

AISLE 1

THE PRODUCE BINS

T*ching, tching, tching.* "Cucumbers, Cantaloupes, 'Taters and 'Maters," *tching, tching.* My childhood summers were filled with the music of not only the bell on the ice cream truck but also of the tinkling necklace of bells worn by the horse (that's right, a horse!) that pulled the cart of the local huckster, our neighborhood produce supplier. This music provided a rhythmic background to the gentleman's bellows as he announced the day's fresh selections. Although my Granny Toni managed to grow a great deal of her own food, she would hail him down when she was running low on staples like onions or potatoes, or wanted to treat us to some of the sweet corn that had come in a bit sooner than hers.

Granny was all business as she surveyed the cart's display of fruits and vegetables on offer from the Eastern Shore farms just a two hour drive away. She peppered the huckster with questions about what had been picked when and the timing of upcoming crops. While the transaction did not make her dig too deeply into her change purse, she was careful with her pennies and intended on spending them wisely. I, on the other hand, was just happy to drink it all in. To have a visit with my bell-wearing friend and get a taste of the melon, cut open and on display, or sample a delicious, ripe strawberry. That's how we got our produce—from the ground or from the cart—all summer long.

I'm not a hundred years old and Granny Toni didn't live in the country. It was the early 1970s and we could see the coal piers of South Baltimore from the top of her street. Yet these invaluable produce providers made their rounds in her neighborhood and others like it to bring the farm to our doorstep. It was a great system: The food was sparklingly fresh, it was local, and it kept area farmers in business.

INDUSTRIAL AGRICULTURE SNAPSHOT

The ring of the bells on that horse now seems like a distant memory. Visits from the huckster have been replaced for most of his customers by visits to the MegaMart, where the dynamic of purchasing produce couldn't be more different. Under the dim flicker of the fluorescent overheads, one doesn't get field reports on the yin and yang of the harvest—which crops are having a good run this season and which might not be. There is no talk of the local weather, the heat wave that has withered the lettuce but sweetened the tomatoes.

Instead there are just row upon row of gleaming waxed fruits and veggies, all lined up like beauty contestants vying for a place in the cart. From a distance, this abundance could be interpreted as a great step forward. Grocery shelves across the nation groan under the weight of pyramids of all manner of fruits and vegetables from the world over, any time of year.

But when I waft a pepper under my nose searching for the smell of garden and am denied that distinct perfume, I know that though these veggies may look pretty enough, they are merely shadows of what they could be.

Ready-for-the-teacher, smooth-skinned apples look great on the shelves. But take one bite and you might as well be eating the decorative wax fruits these perfect specimens so closely resemble (and practically outlast). Berries and stone fruits—once luscious summer luxuries that sweetened the rewards of the ice cream churn—now vie for shelf space year round. But strawberries that taste of cardboard and softball-sized peaches so hard they would be more at home rounding bases than at the dessert table are more the rule than the exception in the produce aisle these days. We can have any food at any time, but is that a good thing?

Productive, uniform, durable. You would think that I was talking about widgets. In fact, I am describing the production goals of industrialized agriculture. A system that has traded taste and texture for ballbearing-like uniformity. Assembly line practices, bedrock to our nation's success in industry, are proving an ill-conceived foundation for our food system. Plants are doused with chemicals before, during, and often after growing to ensure "saleable," picture-perfect produce and to extend their shelf life. Toxic inputs designed to grow everything faster and larger piggyback their way into your crisper drawer. And shortsighted farming practices and government policy are robbing the land of its fertility and farmers and their workers of a living.

Productivity

FERTILITY

It all comes down to dirt. You sweep it out of your house, wash it off of everything from your hands to your dog to your car, and you probably don't think very highly of it. But call it by another name—soil—and you are talking about the foundation of life itself, the mystical medium that can mix with water and sunlight to produce food.

Since ancient times, growers have worshipped, protected, and encouraged the soil's productive ability, its fertility. The tradition of nurturing the soil can be traced back thousands of years to growers such as Asian rice farmers who stocked their paddies with fish that ate crop-depleting pests and deposited mineral-rich fertilizer. American settlers were taught by Native Americans to plant fish heads in their cornfields and to rotate their crops to ensure plentiful yields. And as recently as the last one hundred years, farmers in the Northeast were still sprinkling their fields with oyster shells that supplied a cheap, local source of calcium and other micronutrients to their crops.[1] And when they needed it, these farmers allowed their fields to go unplanted for several seasons so they could rejuvenate before the farmers would sow in them again.

In just a handful of decades, however, the philosophy of fertility has shifted dramatically. Industrial growers have moved from a system that encouraged the development and protection of fertile soil to a system in which the soil is merely the stuff that holds the plant up, and "fertility" is applied from a bag or sprayer. The application of chemical fertilizers became commonplace after World War II. Farmers in the United States more than tripled the amount of chemical fertilizers they used between 1940 and 1965.[2] Pesticides, herbicides, and fungicides completed the arsenal of weapons that industrial farms began to use to combat nature and promote high yields.

Productivity points to one of the many catch-22 scenarios of industrial agriculture. Its practices can lead to an initial increase in production levels, which makes it look like a cure-all to farming's ups and downs, but at the end of the day these methods take more than they give. While some of the impact of these modern practices, such as contamination of the water supply, has already become apparent, other ramifications, like their effect on human health, have yet to be fully realized.

RESIDUES IN THE FOOD SUPPLY, RESIDUES IN OUR BODIES

A portion of the chemical inputs—the fertilizers, pesticides, herbicides, and fungicides—used before, during, and after harvest make their way into your grocery cart and onto your dinner plate.[3] Lists of ingredients are a common sight in the market but are not often seen in the produce aisle— an apple contains just an apple, right? Truth be told, if you are purchasing industrially produced fruits and vegetables, you are taking home a lot more than meets the eye.

Agribusiness would have you believe that chemical inputs are part and parcel of the growing process—so essential that the question no longer remains, "Should there be chemical residue in the food supply?" but is now "How much residue can we tolerate?" The answer to this question can be unclear. There is an ongoing debate surrounding the toxicity of compounds used to grow our produce and the "safe" amounts to ingest. The FDA and the EPA, the government agencies consumers look to for oversight in these areas, are often at loggerheads as to who has jurisdiction over the answers. As a result, these important issues are often unresolved as they get batted back and forth between governing bodies.

Some of the most toxic and environmentally damaging chemicals have been banned from use after decades of heavy applications in the fields. Take the chemical DDT (dichlorodiphenyltrichloroethane), for instance. It gained popularity around the time of World War II when it was developed for use as a pesticide to protect troops from infectious bug bites and was widely applied after the war as an agricultural pesticide. In 1962, Rachel Carson's *Silent Spring* called attention to the vast environmental damage the chemical was causing, but it took ten years for DDT to eventually be banned from the fields for causing reproductive problems, neurological dysfunction, and possibly cancer.[4] And DDT is not alone. There is a running list of chemicals, such as atrazine, one of the nation's most widely used weed killers, that have been linked to human health concerns yet remain in use while under investigation.

Even if a chemical is eventually banned for use in the United States, eaters may still be exposed to it. While farmers aren't using the product, chemical companies are still allowed to produce it. The toxic compounds are then exported to other countries where they continue to be applied to fields. American eaters are exposed to the residues of these banned chemicals when they eat products that have been shipped back to our tables through imports.

Some banned chemicals, such as DDT, have proven to be PBTs (Persistent Bioaccumulative and Toxic Chemicals) that linger in the environment. According to the EPA, PBTs "pose risks to human health and ecosystems. The biggest concerns about PBTs are that they transfer rather easily among air, water, and land, and span boundaries of programs, geography, and generations."[5] Essentially what that means is that chemicals in this group do not break down readily—they remain in the soil and water and are passed along the food chain. Animals ingest PBTs like DDT when they eat plants that are grown in soil or are irrigated by water that contains residues of the chemical. Humans ingest PBT residues by eating such plants, or by eating meat from the animals that grazed on them. All animals, even humans, can pass residues to their young through breast milk. As a result, even though DDT has been banned for more than thirty years, it still shows up in detectable amounts in our food supply and in our bloodstreams.

There seems to be no formal and consistent testing protocol for agricultural compounds. The testing that exists is often conducted or sponsored by the companies that produce the chemicals.[6] And often there is no testing of the effects these chemicals have when used in combination, which is standard practice among growers. Yet, eaters are continually told that the side order of chemicals that comes with their food is "safe." A study by Warren P. Porter, a University of Wisconsin–Madison professor of zoology and environmental toxicology, found that even chemicals such as herbicides, which are widely regarded as benign, can have an impact on immune, endocrine, and nervous system functions when they are consumed in combination with nitrate, a common chemical in fertilizer.[7]

"Safe" residue levels—the amount of a compound that the human body is believed to be able to process without negative impact—are based on averages. The average diet, the average eater, and the average amount of residue found in random samples. But who's average? What if I have a craving for strawberries and eat the whole pint? If I am eating more than an "average" serving I may be poisoning myself.

Children are particularly at risk. Toxic exposure for them is much easier to come by than you might think. In just over every dozen apples, there is one fruit whose level of pesticide is such that eating only half of it would exceed a two-year-old's daily safe exposure limit.[8] Because children eat more food for their body weight than adults, the "average" levels that have been determined for the "average" adult eater are much too high for children.

Uniformity

Some of the most toxic applications to edible plants are not used to increase productivity but are employed for superficial gain alone. Large-scale potato farmers, for example, often apply some of the most dangerous chemicals, such as Monitor, to protect the appearance of the spud—if the potato has brown spots it will only bring minimal dollar from the processor.[9] Uniformity is that highly valued. Tom Pavich, a grower in the San Joaquin Valley of California, told me the story of a retailer who demanded uniformly lime-green grapes—a sure sign of immaturity. Tom said, "We like to have them with a little straw color, a little light banana color—not dark orange, but that turning color. That's when you capture that flavor and the best level of sweetness. And as a result of that the most nutrients, the most antioxidants, the most phytochemicals, and all the things that are good in food. But we were prevented from doing that."

But think snowflakes, autumn leaves. They're more similar than they are different, yet it is their differences that we value. That's the way nature works. Unfortunately, being different is not a feature that industrial agriculture promotes. The size, shape, and rate of the ripening of our produce are closely controlled through intensive breeding programs and the application of additional chemical agents. Unfortunately, the resulting loss of diversity weakens the individual farm and dilutes the food supply.

LACK OF BIODIVERSITY
On the farm, biodiversity applies to the following: 1) genetic diversity, different varieties of the same species such as Macoun, Empire, and Pippin

apples, 2) crop diversity, interplanting a variety of fruits and/or vegetables, and 3) a balanced ecosystem, a synergistic variety of plants, animals, and insects on the farm. They all contribute to a more robust farm that requires less artificial support, such as chemical applications, to thrive.

Genetic diversity is nature's defense mechanism against extinction. It's an evolutionary system that generates a rainbow of subtle differences within a plant species. In the 1400s, the Incas used it to their advantage in the cultivation of potatoes. They raised thousands of different varieties, each a variation on the potato theme that bore a unique level of pest resistance, nutrient use, drought tolerance, and overall nutritional benefit. In doing so, farmers could hedge their bets against the entire harvest being destroyed. The varying strengths of the different potato varieties guaranteed that blight from pests, disease, or weather might eliminate some of the varieties some of the time but wouldn't be able to take down all of the varieties at any time.

Crop diversity, also called intercropping, planting different crops on neighboring fields or within the same field, also provides a barrier of defense against the elements. For example, variations in weather conditions, if not natural-disaster-extreme, are better absorbed by plants of differing needs—one drought-tolerant, one less susceptible to being waterlogged. Or, low-growing ground cover can be interplanted with taller crops to promote water retention and contribute to soil nutrition. Changing the arrangement of crops every few harvests also helps eliminate pests, which often take several seasons to infest a field.

Planting different crops in close proximity can also encourage a balanced ecosystem within the farm. Worms, for example, aerate the soil with their wiggling and enrich it with their castings. Pollinators like bees are often essential to healthy crops. Insects such as ladybugs, as cute as they might be, are also voracious eaters of plant-destroying aphids and can be released in fields to greatly eliminate the need for artificial pesticide application. The borders of fields are often planted with flowering growth, which contributes to biodiversity by providing shelter for all of these hardworking friends of the farm and pest-devouring winged workers, such as bats and birds.

When these three levels of biodiversity—genetic, crop, and ecosystem—are reduced, so is the resilience of the farm. I'm not speaking about "could happens" here; it did happen. Between 1846 and 1850, the Irish Potato Famine was responsible for the deaths of about one million citizens and caused a mass emigration from Ireland. It was triggered by a lack of genetic and crop diversity—the country was planted largely with one kind of potato on which the poor relied almost entirely for food. A rogue fungus invaded and destroyed the crop, leaving this segment of the population without a thing to eat and the country in dire straits.

While we are not at risk of starving in a single season now, industrial farming practices have put our food supply in an unstable position. Genetic diversity has been indiscriminately reduced. The varieties of fruits and vegetables grown commercially and available at the MegaMart are a small fraction of the diversity that was cultivated before the age of industrial agriculture. Fruits such as the Fiesta and Pink Pearl apples that our forefathers snacked on have disappeared from orchards in favor of the ubiquitous, but often bland varieties such as Red Delicious.[10] This didn't happen by chance. There was no agricultural ice age that wiped them out like so many dinosaurs. Agribusiness has whittled down the assortment of fruits and vegetables that are grown to a handful of standardized varieties that fit into automated processes. Plants that are too delicate to withstand the toxic applications of chemicals, the rough hands of mechanized cultivation and harvest, and the many miles of travel from farm to table have fallen into obscurity or have gone extinct in favor of predictable, machine-friendly produce.

These limited varieties are then planted on huge swaths of acreage, eliminating crop diversity and replacing it with monoculture farming. Dousing the fields with pesticides deals the final blow, eliminating beneficial insects from the ecosystem and throwing it off balance. The result is weak crops propped up on the flimsy crutches of agriculture chemicals to support their growth.

DEVELOPMENT OF GENETICALLY MODIFIED ORGANISMS (GMOs)

Until recently, GMO research has concentrated mainly on the modification of cereal crops such as corn and soy, but the focus is sharpening on the genetic manipulation of fruits and vegetables to obtain predictable, uniform produce. As I'll discuss in Aisle 4: Grains, Oils, and Sweeteners, there are many concerns surrounding the planting of GMO crops.

Paramount among these concerns is the threat GMOs pose to biodiversity. Some fear that, like the mass plantings of the Green Revolution of the 1960s, which replaced indigenous crops with plants that were highly dependent on first-world technologies such as chemical fertilizers and pesticides, farming GMO crops will wipe out native crops and decimate the genetic diversity of the world's plant supply.

Others fear health consequences, and such fears are not unfounded. The Flavr Savr tomato, developed by Calgene, Inc., was introduced into the market as a more "transportable" tomato that could be shipped longer distances and lasted longer on the shelf. It was eventually pulled from markets in 1997 after several reports linked consumption of the tomatoes to the development of stomach lesions.[11]

Durability

TRANSPORTATION

Whether it's getting an item from point A to point B, or extending its shelf life, durability has been a driving force behind the push for uniformity and is a critical component in agribusiness. Fruits and vegetables are built to travel, look good on the shelf, and stay pretty for the longest time—flavor is not a priority. Whether it's by rail, truck, or airplane, fruits and vegetables clock a lot of miles. The typical American meal travels on average 1,500 to 2,500 miles from place of origin to your plate.[12] No matter where in the United States you live, nine months out of the year most of the fruits and vegetables that you eat come from California.[13]

Beyond the California season, the majority of our fruits and vegetables are imported. If you are eating a melon in January, chances are it's from Mexico, or points beyond, as are many of the items in the produce aisle during the dead of winter when even California gets chilly. It takes a lot of fuel to transport these out-of-season items to your area MegaMart. Buy a lot of such items and you are loading up your grocery cart with as much fuel as fruits and vegetables.

EXTENDED GROWING SEASON AND SHELF LIFE

Many industrial growers go to great lengths to artificially extend their growing season. Orange growers in the San Joaquin Valley in California spray trees with gibberellic acid and another compound called 2,4-D to delay maturity, and to stretch their growing season.[14] Not surprisingly, however, the very factors that promote the fruit's ubiquitous presence on the shelf often degrade its quality.[15]

Tomatoes are typically harvested unripe so that their hard flesh is easier to ship. They are then treated with ethylene gas, which imbues them with the fire-engine red color we expect to give contrast to our salads. The result is the mealy specimen that looks great but tastes awful. And it's not just tomatoes; oranges, mangoes, bananas, and peaches are just a few of the items in the produce aisle that are treated in this manner.

Ethylene gas in and of itself is not harmful. It is a naturally occurring organic vapor that you can generate at home by putting a bunch of green bananas in a paper bag. But when it is used in the commercial environment, it robs the fruits and vegetables of their opportunity to deliver the most flavor and nutrients when you cut into them. As a matter of fact, a Cornell University study has recognized that force-ripened produce is less nutritious than ripe-harvested crops.[16] At the end of the day, it's all about return on investment. You get out what you put in. And I would rather be eating a "veggie bank" full of sunshine and rainwater than one that was pumped full of ripening gas.

In addition to "gassing," a number of methods are employed to keep the produce appealing to the eye while it bides its time on the shelf.

GAS EXCHANGE Advancements in packaging have allowed an influx of bagged lettuces to flood the market. The bags that contain your spring mix often use gas-exchange technology to keep the blush on the bloom, so to speak. "Breathable" plastic bags and injections of gases such as nitrogen slow the rotting process. But by the time these lettuces are washed, processed, shipped, and stocked, they can be more than two weeks old.[17]

FUNGICIDAL WAXES To fend off the course of nature, vendors often spray items like cucumbers, peppers, and apples with fungicidal waxes. If you've ever picked up a potential pickle and it felt sort of oily in your hand, you know what I'm talking about. Waxes are applied to delay spoilage by reducing moisture loss and forming a physical barrier against contamination.

WRAPPERS The tissue of individually wrapped fruits and vegetables is often impregnated with fungicides and bactericides to extend shelf life.

COLD STORAGE While there is no other tomato like that which is plucked from the vine and eaten, having never known the inside of a cooler box, it is a pleasure that few ever know. Which is too bad, because to keep tomatoes tasty, they should never be refrigerated. While cold storage is a viable preservative for some produce items, such as potatoes, apples, and carrots (think root cellar), it wreaks havoc on others. I hate to feel a cold tomato or see an ear of corn break out into a sweat because of its shift from the cooler to the display shelf. These types of produce suffer under refrigeration—it turns their sweet sugars into flavorless starch.

REVIVING REAL FOOD

Farming wasn't meant to be this way. As Hall Gibson, a farmer in Brewster, New York, explains, "Farming should work in concert with nature, not against it." He is one of many farmers who are building an alternative food supply for eaters who value the many benefits of growing in harmony with nature. (Hall is profiled on page 37.)

Farmers like Hall don't want to turn the clock back, but they aren't afraid to borrow a page from their grandfather's growing manual (sometimes, in fact, they *are* the grandfathers) and revisit the sustainable practices that have successfully fed eaters until recently. Not only do they reduce or eliminate the use of toxic chemicals on their land, they also work to conserve water and soil by planting cover crops that form a retentive web over their fields, protect beneficial insects, and break down to nourish the soil. They rotate crops, plant crop borders, and allow fields to go unplanted for a time to provide habitat for indigenous wildlife, preserving biodiversity. They practice IPM (integrated pest management) that, while not always completely chemical-free, works in harmony with the local ecosystem to promote crop health.

Many of these farmers are part grower, part inventor/innovator. For example, farming pioneer Eliot Coleman is using greenhouses to extend the growing season, with no negative impact to the environment or reduction in the quality of the produce. While operating a greenhouse, also referred to as a hothouse, used to consume a lot of energy, design advancements have progressed greatly and they can now be used year round without being heated. At his place in Maine, Eliot has designed a system of buildings that not only harness the heat of even the dim rays of the winter's sun but, because of the tightly controlled conditions, efficiently yield bumper crops on a small fraction of the acreage of an outdoor field.

Cabbage Hill Farm in Mount Kisco, New York, is the site of another exercise in innovation. They operate an aquaponics system, a combination of aquaculture (raising fish) and hydroponics (raising vegetables in a liquid medium rather than dirt) that demonstrates some exciting advances in sustainability. The term hydroponic sometimes has a negative connotation, referring to plants raised in a chemically saturated potting medium. The aquaponics technique, on the other hand, recirculates nutrient-rich water from the fish tanks to nourish and grow the lettuce beds. No chemicals are used—they would kill the fish. The health of the system relies on maintaining a level of beneficial bacteria and introducing measured amounts of salt when there is evidence of illness. The vegetarian tilapia are fed a pellet food, but Cabbage Hill is working with feed companies to develop an organic supply. Local chefs, market owners, and eaters alike enjoy the tender leaves and impeccably fresh fish that are abundant year round.

Innovation would be hollow, however, if it didn't provide the desired result, which for farmers interested in sustainability is, in large part, flavor. They do what they do to recapture and secure the diverse spectrum of flavorful foods once available to us. Here are some strategies for locating and identifying the tastiest and purest fruits and vegetables.

Buy Local, Buy Seasonal

This is really the mantra of good eating and a recurrent theme of this book. It is the only way to experience fruits and vegetables at their full potential. Local, seasonal produce looks, smells, tastes, sounds, and feels ripe and ready to eat, fulfilling all of the senses.

But how do you know what's in season? It can be easy to forget that even items such as green beans will only have their characteristic snap during part of the year or that apples lose their crunch over time. If you favor a scholastic approach, you can contact your state's Department of Agriculture for a Produce Availability chart. Most have them posted on their Web site (just use a search engine for "[insert state] Department of Agriculture" to locate their Web address). Then you can use it to buy items that are only in season in your area. The more closely you keep to it, the more delicious the possibilities in the kitchen will be.

Perhaps the easiest and most pleasurable way to enjoy delicious, sustainable, seasonal eating is to buy local. Why? For reasons both logical and less so. On the objective side of the argument, because the net environmental impact is less—products that haven't been shipped thousands of miles haven't paid a price in fossil fuel. And if my fruit is coming from down the street rather than from around the globe, it will require fewer "freshness" enhancers to keep it looking pretty for a longer time.

But an even greater draw for me is the subjective list of pros. From a culinary point of view, since it hasn't had to withstand the rigor of travel, a local item has been picked closer to peak ripeness so it will provide me with more flavor, better texture, and possibly more nutrients. And, aesthetically speaking, the local fruit is my vote for a landscape that is dotted with agrarian views. I want the caretaking of land and feeding of my community to remain a part of my culture—not a centralized and distant commodity.

You don't have to be maniacal about eating local, just mindful. For example, I don't know about you but I cannot go all winter without a single B.L.T. sandwich. Even though I know my "L" has probably seen enough of the road to qualify for its own AAA card, and my "T" is bringing more moisture than flavor to the party, I need the sandwich and I know my "B" will mask the veggies' deficiencies. I wouldn't, however, even consider whipping up a batch of gazpacho in January or give in to my craving for homemade salsa on Super Bowl Sunday because I know it's just not going to happen tastewise. These dishes rely too heavily on the star players—the tomatoes—and there is no way I am going to get the big tomato flavor out of a winterized version of the fruit. Nor am I willing to invest that heavily in imports for something that will come around if I'm just a little patient. I have to wait until it's summer in my area again, when tomatoes are heavy on the vine. Then it's "Viva la salsa!"

Buy Directly from the Producer

Sometimes it can be a challenge to find local produce in the MegaMart. Often small farmers are locked out of the current distribution system, designed to work on economies of scale. But while everyone may not have a cattle ranch in their neighborhood or live on the coast with easy access to the daily catch, nearly everyone in the United States can get their hands on delicious, nonindustrial produce.

Buying directly from the farmer benefits both the grower and the eater. Many of the farms that sell directly to consumers are family-owned and operated and are struggling to remain so. They can't afford to pay for third-party marketing and distribution. Others aren't willing to conform to the narrow, and many would say lower, "freshness" guidelines for durability and uniformity that large distributors require.

But for many farmers, the decision to sell directly to their eaters is more than a business strategy. After all, food is personal. And the connection between growers and eaters that develops over a direct exchange goes beyond a monetary transaction, particularly regarding food that's raised with care and attention. For the eater, the food tastes better when you know where it comes from and how it was raised, and you value it more when you've shaken the hand that produced it. For the growers, selling the highest quality items directly to the eater closes the circle of a food chain to which these farmers are highly dedicated.

And the quality does shine through. You are buying food about as close to its source as possible. So it hasn't spent days in shipping and receiving and hasn't been picked unripe to keep it from bruising in transit. It is harvested impeccably fresh, often the morning that you pick it up.

You can also learn a lot by talking directly with your grower—about their production methods as well as the items they have on offer. Growers often will gladly share cooking tips on any unusual items such as ramps, purslane, or fiddlehead ferns. Or give you ideas for old standards—corn, potatoes, carrots—so you can mix it up a bit. They can let you know what will be ripe in the coming weeks so you can plan ahead. Some even distribute newsletters, such as the *Ladybug Letter* published by Mariquita Farms in Northern California, to keep their eaters informed on all of these fronts.

A relationship with your grower is particularly valuable if you have children. Details such as "broccoli doesn't grow on trees" and that there is a face—the farmer's—behind every bite on their plate are valuable lessons that can inform kids' eating. Local newspapers often list farms where children can take a basket out to Pick-Your-Own, drink cider from a real mill, or maybe learn how to milk a cow. Some direct buying programs invite members onto the farm to participate in the planting, weeding, and harvesting. What kid doesn't enjoy an opportunity to dig in the dirt or unearth a couple of worms? They won't even notice that they are getting an education about their food in the process. After a day of planting, harvesting, or just romping, they may even voluntarily eat something green.

And sometimes direct-to-buyer farms act in larger ways, too, helping the community beyond providing a market for fresh food—in New Jersey, the Youth Farmstand Project employs at-risk youths at farmstands across the state. The kids learn valuable business lessons and experience what it's like to be an integral, positive part of a community.

Here are three ways you can buy directly from the farmer:

FARMERS' MARKETS

I can't imagine a worse way to spend a sunny afternoon than at the Mega-Mart pushing around a cart the size of a minivan under fluorescent, soul-stealing lights. Shopping at the farmers' market, on the other hand, turns a chore into a pleasure. Bushels of fresh picked apples—Jonagolds, Macouns, Pippins—catch your eye. Across the way, a line is growing for farm-fresh eggs, and omelette makers chat with uncharacteristic ease as they wait for their dozen. Bouquets of fresh herbs find their way into your tote and perfume your journey. All as you enjoy the passing breeze and chat with growers and fellow eaters.

And because the food of a good market is grown locally, the market gives its visitors a sense of place—it belongs to their region; you can't replicate it quite the same way anywhere else. Plus, you can bring your kids—they'll like it too—and they might even learn a little about the food chain in the process. And all of this joy doesn't end at the market—it will be evident on your dinner plate as well.

When you are looking for a good market, you need to make sure that the producers are the sellers. There are some markets that pick up boxes of goods from the same distributors that serve the MegaMarts, sell them in the open air, and call their markets "farmers' markets." Make sure that you are dealing with the people who actually grow, raise, or craft the food, not distributors. All you have to do is ask anyone attending the stalls if they grew their goods or call the market manager ahead of time to make sure.

Riff-Raff Stew

The versatility of this dish—you can use just about any kind of vegetables that you have on hand to whip it up—makes it easy to incorporate whatever fresh produce you find at the market. The secret ingredient, the Parmesan rind, brings a lot of hearty flavor to the dish.

3 tablespoons olive oil
1 large onion, diced
1 teaspoon salt, plus more to taste
½ teaspoon freshly ground black pepper, plus more to taste
4 garlic cloves, chopped
1 bunch greens such as kale, collard, chard, or spinach, roughly chopped (optional)
1 teaspoon dried thyme, or 1 tablespoon fresh, chopped
1 bay leaf
One 28-ounce can peeled whole tomatoes, crushed
1 quart chicken stock, preferably homemade (see recipe, page 79)
2 cups assorted root vegetables such as potatoes, sweet potatoes, carrots, or turnips, peeled and diced into 1-inch cubes
Rind from a wedge of Parmesan cheese (at least 2 to 3 inches long)
2 to 3 cups assorted vegetable drawer riff-raff (such as a handful of green beans, a sweet pepper, a wedge of cabbage, corn from the cob), cut into bite-size pieces
2 cups white beans or garbanzo beans, preferably slow-cooked (see recipe, page 74), or 2 cups cooked small pasta (optional)
2 ounces grated Parmesan cheese, for serving

Heat the oil in a large Dutch oven or soup pot over medium heat. Add the onion, along with 1 teaspoon salt and ½ teaspoon pepper, and sauté until translucent, 5 to 7 minutes. Add the garlic and sauté until fragrant, about 1 minute. Add the greens, if using, and sauté until wilted. Stir in the thyme and bay leaf, then add the tomatoes and simmer until slightly thickened, 5 to 7 minutes. Add the chicken stock, root vegetables, and cheese rind and simmer until the vegetables are almost tender, about 15 minutes. Add the riff-raff and simmer another 10 minutes, or until the root vegetables are very tender. Add the beans or pasta, if using, and heat through. Add salt and pepper to taste. Ladle into serving bowls and sprinkle each with grated cheese.

Serves 4

FARMSTANDS

Across the country, farmstands range from a card table set up at the bottom of the driveway of a farm displaying the morning's egg collection, to much more elaborate setups, boasting Pick-Your-Own fields, petting zoos, piping hot baked goods—even hayrides.

In their own way, farmstands have more in common with a 7-Eleven than they do with a big grocery store. As with the 7-Eleven, when it comes to convenience, nothing could be easier than a farmstand. Simply pull up, hop out, make your selections, and you're on your way. No need for cumbersome shopping carts or the fight for a parking spot in a gigantic lot. Farmstands often flourish in vacation regions, where tourists are hungry for local flavor. If you are traveling in an agricultural area, I can think of no better souvenir than a bushel of the local harvest.

These stands may or may not be attended. I think my favorite farmstand is the kid-run "lemonade stand" type farmstand. I enjoy their budding entrepreneurship and am happy to contribute to their homespun MBA program. It is not entirely uncommon, however, to see an unmanned farmstand, one that operates on an honor system—just a pile of fresh picked produce and a cash can. By all means, if you patronize such a stand, honor the honor system, and maybe even include a tip for good service, so to speak.

COMMUNITY SUPPORTED AGRICULTURE (CSA)

I don't like to garden. Oh, I throw a few plants in a pot every year and have a little collection of herbs and things that are the product of my "rite of spring" gardening frenzy. But after that weekend is over, I'm back in the kitchen and happy to leave the growing to the experts. Last summer, however, I was lured to the toil of the soil by my one holy grail—exquisitely fresh, organic fruits and vegetables. I joined a CSA, a Community Supported (or Sponsored) Agriculture program, run by Ellen and Walter Greist at their Mill River Valley Gardens, in North Haven, Connecticut, and was able to share in the harvest for the duration of the summer and long into the fall.

A CSA is essentially a partnership between the grower and the eater. A CSA grower calculates the carrying capacity of his land—the number of families that it can feed for the season. Eaters pay a lump sum in advance of the harvest to purchase one of these "shares," which entitles them to that fraction of the harvest for the length of the growing season.

Each CSA is unique, so it's important to find one that reflects your values and will fit into your lifestyle. Some are organic, some are not. Many CSAs require members to pick up at the farm, but others have satellite pick-up points that are more centrally located, even in such metropolises as New York. A portion of CSAs have a work requirement—members either spend time in the fields, washing and sorting the harvest, or man the distribution sites. The cost of membership varies, as does the size of the share—many offer half-shares for singles or small families—so shop around to find one that fits the size of your budget and your appetite.

If the idea of paying up front is daunting to you, don't let it keep you from investigating CSA. Many will set up payment programs to help you space out your dues if you need to. Some CSA programs accept food stamps. Others will reduce share costs for an increased work commitment. Programs like Just Food in New York City (www.justfood.org) connect low-income families with CSA farmers who are willing to work on a sliding scale.

CSA is a wonderful way to eat Real Food, but it is a commitment. If you sign up, you need to show up. So be prepared to make arrangements for your weekly pickup if you aren't going to make it—send a friend or split the pickups with a neighbor member so you can take turns making the drive. The worst thing you can do is abandon the food—leave it to wilt in a corner after all of the hard work it has taken to get it eater-ready. (For a CSA Profile, see Kanalani Ohana Farm on page 228.)

HOW TO DO IT
To find farmers' markets, farmstands, and CSAs in your area, you can utilize the following resources:

LOCAL HARVEST
www.localharvest.org
A national search engine for local food sources.

ALTERNATIVE FARMING SYSTEMS INFORMATION CENTER
www.nal.usda.gov/afsic/csa/csastate.htm
The USDA's comprehensive listing of CSA farms.

FARMERS' MARKETS
www.ams.usda.gov/farmersmarkets/map.htm
The USDA maintains an alphabetical directory of farmers' markets organized by state.

ROBYN VAN EN CENTER FOR CSA RESOURCES
www.csacenter.org
Provides support for sustainable agricultural initiatives and has a search engine for locating CSAs.

Indirectly from the Farmer

If you can't get to a farmer, consider finding a trusted third party to help you gather your feast. These alternatives to the MegaMart—the local co-op, independent health food store, and privately owned grocery—are more likely to have direct relationships with small growers. And they often supplement at least some, if not all, of their inventory with locally produced items. For family farmers, particularly those who can't or choose not to sell directly to eaters, such models offer a viable distribution solution for their products. (See Building a Better Grocery Store, page 233, for more information about these third-party resources.)

Consider Organic

On October 21, 2002, the U.S. Department of Agriculture put into effect the National Organic Standards, a set of criteria that must be met for food to be labeled organic. The Standards address many of the issues regarding the use of chemicals in the growing and handling of food, but detractors say these don't go far enough, particularly in the area of environmental protection. While they may not cover all of the bases, the Organic Standards go a long way toward moving the food system away from its intensive use of chemical inputs, and guarantee that you will not be unwittingly eating GMOs.

WHAT IS ORGANIC?

The National Organic Standards, as they apply to fruits and vegetables, guarantee that:

- Produce is grown without the use of most conventional pesticides.
- Produce may not be grown with fertilizers made with synthetic ingredients or sewage sludge.
- Bioengineering (GMOs) is not allowed.

• In a retail environment, produce sold as "organic" must be separated from conventional items during transport, storage, and display to reduce possible contact contamination with chemical residues.

Farms that grow or raise more than $5,000 worth of organic food per year and companies that handle or process organic food must apply for certification to use the term and are inspected by government-approved certifiers to guarantee that they are in compliance with the USDA Organic Standards. All organic food must bear the name of the certifying agent for your reference (for fruits and vegetables that you buy in a grocery, this name comes on the shipping carton so you won't see it on the produce, but it must be provided upon request).

It's important to note that, as public policy, the National Organic Standards are subject to revision. To keep up to date on any changes in the standards or to review the full text of the regulations and policies, visit the Web site for the National Organic Program (NOP) at www.ams.usda.gov/nop/.

LABELING ORGANIC

Organic produce may bear the USDA Organic seal (see below) but such a seal is not required. Often there will be a tiny sticker on fruits and veggies that identifies the food as organic, but it may not include the seal or, in a farmers' market, a grower may just put a sign on top of his bushel that says the food is organic without an illustration of the seal. That's okay. If the word "organic" is displayed, the grower has to be certified and must show proof of certification if you ask for it.

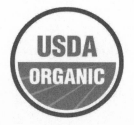

Look Beyond Organic

Even though we now have a National Organic Program, there is no seal or certification that has all of the answers, or that addresses all of the issues involved in eating sustainably. There are a lot of farmers doing great work—even going above and beyond the requirements of the National Organic Program—who are not certified. The process is too expensive for some—there is an annual certification fee and the record keeping is labor intensive—and it is the sole responsibility of the farmer. For some, government involvement and its inherent bureaucracy have taken the spirit out of organic, which began as a grassroots movement fueled by an appreciation for natural resources and unadulterated foods. They argue that the National Organic Program, with its cumbersome paperwork and loopholes, is suited for big businesses that can easily absorb the time and money spent on certification. They believe the National Organic Program has paved the way for "industrial organic" farmers—large operations that swap out toxic chemical inputs for less noxious ones, but still follow industrial practices that ignore important environmental and social issues.

How do you know if a farmer's practices go beyond organic? While there are a smattering of seals in development, there is no black and white answer, no seal that covers all of the bases. The only way to know is to talk with the grower, or with a co-op owner or market manager you trust who has a relationship with the farmer. It all comes down to the human connection that has become lost in the current agricultural model. I don't want food that is grown by machine, and one of the best ways to avoid that is to meet the pair of hands that are doing the growing themselves.

Other Seals

Consumer demand for organic produce and farmers' dissatisfaction with organic certification criteria have led to a host of eco-labels—claims that a product has a certain ecological benefit—entering the marketplace. Consumers Union, a consumer advocacy group that publishes *Consumer Reports* magazine, does a good job of assessing a variety of eco-labels. They evaluate them on the meaning of the label, the consistency of the certification process, the public availability of its certification criteria and names of its board members, the process for developing the label, and any potential conflict of interest in its development or use. Their Web site, www.eco-labels.org, is updated frequently to keep their label assessments current and includes new labels as they hit the shelves.

Support Family Farmers

I will always throw my support behind the efforts of the dedicated people who are trying to maintain an agrarian tradition in this country in the face of the cultural, political, and economic forces working against them. I don't want to see organic go the same way as our current agricultural system—owned by a few conglomerates who are more interested in (or are behind) the latest food craze than they are in producing quality food. It is more important to support a family-owned and -operated farm that honors the land and community but may not be certified organic than it is to purchase certified organic produce from halfway around the world.

Shop for Taste, Not Appearance

The old joke goes, "What's worse than seeing a worm in your apple? Seeing half a worm." I would say the worst is seeing no worm at all. Not to say that you should be eating a salad of pest-ridden delicacies, but don't be afraid of seeing the occasional critter in your pile of Granny Smiths (or better yet, your heirloom Macouns) or peeking out from the silk of a fresh ear of corn. They're your guarantee that your food is part of the circle of life and hasn't been doused out of the realm of nature by a confluence of chemicals. And if it isn't good enough for a worm, it shouldn't be good enough for you, either.

Fruits and vegetables shouldn't look like they've been pressed out of an assembly line template. Subtle variations in size, shape, and color aren't just okay; that's how they are meant to be. That Quasimodo-looking tomato may not be the prettiest belle at the ball, but it just very well may be the tastiest. Think of it as proof that your produce has lived a life and has built some character along the way.

Ugly Tomato Pie

This easy dish is especially good for those end-of-summer, enormous, often misshapen tomatoes—they're not especially pretty, but they pack marvelous taste.

1 recipe Basic Pie Dough, defrosted if frozen (recipe follows)
2 large "ugly" tomatoes, sliced into ½-inch rounds (you should have about 10 slices)
1 cup grated Gruyère cheese
1 cup fresh basil, torn into pieces

Preheat the oven to 350°F. Press the pie dough into a 9-inch pie pan and prick all over with a fork. Bake for 10 minutes, or until partially cooked through and just beginning to turn golden. Meanwhile, place the tomato slices on paper towels and let sit for 10 minutes to absorb excess juices. When the pie crust is ready, sprinkle a third of the cheese on the bottom of the crust, followed by half the tomato slices, overlapping slightly. Sprinkle half the basil over the top. Press down lightly with the back of a spoon. Repeat layers of cheese, tomato slices, and basil, ending with the rest of the cheese. Return to the oven and bake for 30 minutes, or until golden brown and bubbly on top. Cool for 10 minutes before serving, or serve at room temperature.

Serves 6

BASIC PIE DOUGH

1⅓ cups all-purpose flour
1 stick (½ cup) salted butter, chilled
¼ cup ice water

Place the flour in a food processor fitted with the metal blade. Slice the butter into the flour and process until the mixture resembles coarse cornmeal. Then slowly pour the water into the feed tube. Process until the mixture comes together and forms a ball. Dough can be frozen if desired; wrap closely in plastic wrap, place in a plastic bag, and freeze until ready to use.

Makes dough for one 9-inch crust

Heirloom varieties, which are grown for taste, not durability, may look like nothing you've ever seen. But if you come across them, you've hit the jackpot. Speckled beans, purple potatoes, bicolored tomatoes might look like they are from outer space, but they are just a fraction of the rainbow of varieties that offer big flavor.

While there is no precise definition for heirloom produce, the term is used in the agricultural community to describe noncommercial, nonhybridized plants that are bred to continue a valued species line. Farmers who grow heirloom products are the real heroes of genetic diversity, protecting varieties that would otherwise go extinct in the industrial farming system. The fruits and vegetables are raised for taste and quality, and often have a rich history that can be traced back across generations of farmers. Their names, often lyrical (Listada de Gandia eggplants, Pruden's Purple tomatoes) and otherwise descriptive (Burpless Muncher cucumbers) are often as complex as their flavors.

Because heirloom crops rarely provide the cookie-cutter uniformity or fast growing properties of commercial varieties they have traditionally been the dominion of the home gardener or family farmer. However, the taste benefits of heirloom items have caught the eyes of chefs and diners alike, and they are increasingly available on restaurant menus. Their quality is so superior when compared to commercially raised products that it is not uncommon for a chef to contract with a family farm to have heirloom items raised to order. Chances are, if you are buying directly from the farmer—at the farmers' market, a farmstand, or through a CSA—you are already enjoying heirloom varieties, as many conscious growers prefer to plant these exciting specimens.

Use Your Nose

When I walk through the produce aisle I look like a hound dog. I could never figure out that thumping thing; when I want a good cantaloupe I give it a whiff—"Ahh, summer." Other good candidates for the sniff test include lemons, limes, oranges, peaches, and even tomatoes, which should smell of the vine. Try it and I bet you will be able to do half of your shopping with your eyes closed.

Avoid Highly Toxic Foods

The Environmental Working Group lists twelve fruits and vegetables in the supermarket aisles that have the highest levels of chemical residues. They suggest that by eliminating these foods, an eater can reduce his or her total dietary risk from pesticides by 50 percent. Alternative produce selections are also listed. Both lists are kept current and are available on their Web site, www.ewg.org.[18]

Eat a Variety of Fruits and Vegetables

This is the best way of spreading out your potential risks. By eating a variety of items, you won't continually be exposing yourself to any toxic chemicals that are used to grow that particular variety.

PLU Codes

Those little stickers on your produce aren't just ads. The digits on fruits and vegetables can be helpful. Produce bearing codes that begin in 9 is organic, and codes that begin in 8 are genetically modified (see page 118 for a discussion of genetically modified organisms).

Make Your Own Bagged Vegetables

When you buy bagged items, like salad mixes or those whittled down carrot nibs, you are paying for a lot more than the vegetables. The packaging technology relies on complex and costly machinery that must be constantly updated to stay ahead of the competitive curve. Teams of workers are needed to handle the product—all of which you pay for with your grocery dollars. The fuel to run the machinery and the shipping to get the produce from harvest to processing plants increase the costs to you and the impact on the environment. Additionally, small farmers who cannot afford this capital-intensive infrastructure are priced out of business.

Opt instead for minimally packaged items like bundled lettuces. When you get them home, wash them in a sink full of cold water, spin them to thoroughly dry, and store them, wrapped in damp paper towels and sealed in a (reusable) Ziploc bag, in your crisper drawer. The same holds for carrots and other snackable crudite. Peeled, washed, and cut into chunks, these items will stay bright for several days using the same damp paper towel system.

Scrub It

You see the message everywhere: "Wash all fruits and vegetables thoroughly." This applies to all produce, organic or conventional. Organic farmers use composted manure as fertilizer, and you want to make sure you wash off any traces of that. And, although organic produce may not be raised with pesticides, it may have picked up some residue on its way to you, so you want to get rid of that, too.

A good washing, no matter how thorough, will not remove all of the chemicals from industrially raised produce. Some applications are systemic—absorbed into the cell walls of the food as it grows. Others are petroleum-based, so a rinse under the faucet won't break these applications down. To remove as much residue as possible, you don't need a special "veggie wash." Just swish items with edible peels like apples and peaches in a small bowl of warm water and a few drops of fragrance-free soap and rinse thoroughly.

Peel It

Peeling is another way to limit your exposure to agricultural chemicals. While not all chemical applications are on the surface of the plants, a lot are. It's also important to scrub the surfaces of items like melons and oranges that you intend to hollow or peel to prevent any residues that might dissolve in the juices of these fruits from winding up on your cutting board or your plate. Peel or remove the outer leaves from items like lettuce before washing.

Can It, Dry It, Freeze It

The laws of supply and demand often kick in when fruits and vegetables are in peak season, so you can stretch your grocery budget further. And if you really want to take advantage of the lower prices that accompany the season's bounty, then freeze, can, and dry everything you're able to and you'll be stocked until the next season. You can have berries in January—just pull out your jar of jam or enjoy your frozen ones, sugared and heated until bubbling, on just about anything. Herbs can be cleaned, chopped, and added to ice cube trays partially filled with water—add to winter dishes for a taste of summer freshness.

And then there's the occasional bumper crop—the zucchini that just kept coming or the farmer's "experimental" crop that just happened to be perfectly suited for the land and gave forth in unexpected abundance. Such bounty forces you to come up with interesting ways to utilize the embarrassment of riches. And if you run out of ideas, you can always freeze it.

Grilled Veggie Hero with Roasted Garlic Spread

This sandwich is great for using up some of the bounty from the farmers' market. The hours that it spends wrapped in plastic make this a terrific dish for entertaining or to take on a picnic.

1 head garlic
Olive oil for drizzling and brushing
Salt and freshly ground black pepper
2 portobello mushroom caps

2 to 3 zucchini or yellow squash, sliced lengthwise into thirds
1 Vidalia or red onion, thickly sliced crosswise
2 red peppers, cut in half, stems, ribs, and seeds removed
One 7-ounce log goat cheese
2 tablespoons whole milk or sour cream
1 loaf rustic bread such as ciabatta
1 tomato, thinly sliced
2 tablespoons balsamic vinegar
1 bunch arugula or 3 cups fresh spinach, chopped

Preheat the oven to 325°F. Cut off the top quarter of the garlic head to expose the cloves. Drizzle with oil, sprinkle with salt and pepper, and wrap tightly in aluminum foil. Place on a cookie sheet and bake until soft, 45 minutes to 1 hour. Remove from the oven and set aside to cool.

Preheat the broiler. Brush the mushroom caps, zucchini or squash, onion, and peppers with oil and season with salt and pepper. Broil 3 to 4 inches from the element until tender, about 10 minutes, turning once. Set aside to cool.

Squeeze the roasted garlic out of the skin into a small bowl and mash with a fork. Add the goat cheese, milk or sour cream, and salt and pepper to taste, continuing to mash well with a fork until blended.

Cut the bread in half and open it like a book. Spread both sides of the bread with the goat cheese mixture. Slice the roasted vegetables into strips and layer them on one side of bread. Top the vegetables with tomato slices. Drizzle with vinegar. Top with arugula or spinach and replace the top half of the bread to make a sandwich. Press the length of the sandwich firmly with the palm of your hand to compress it slightly. Wrap tightly in plastic wrap and press under a weight (2 cans of tomatoes on top of a cutting board works well) for 2 to 3 hours to combine the flavors and improve the sandwich texture. Cut into portions and serve.

Serves 6 as part of a picnic buffet

NOTE: The vegetables can be grilled a day ahead and the roasted garlic spread can be made up to 2 days ahead and stored in the refrigerator.

Buy Dried, Canned, or Frozen

When fruits and vegetables are out of season, but you would still like them in your diet, opt for dried, canned, and frozen items over shipped and imported fresh ones. Of these three types of preserved products, dried are the easiest on the environment; they are light, so they don't rack up as much petroleum in transport as heavy canned items and, unlike frozen fruits and vegetables, they don't require costly refrigeration in transport, at the market, and in your kitchen.

Grow a Little Something

I have a really black thumb. I am notorious for my "Addams family" garden, a gothic collection of dead plants that were going to be my culinary herb garden but are now an assembly of plant skeletons in artfully arranged containers in a corner of my kitchen.

Fortunately, there are gifted growers out there who have been willing to trade skills with me. When I lived in Manhattan, my neighbor shared with me a bountiful harvest of tomatoes that she grew in pots on her fire escape. In exchange I turned her donation into fresh salsa and we enjoyed it with tortilla chips and some margaritas.

If you have a spare corner, a little sunlight, and even a brown thumb, give growing a try. If you're not successful, you can always hook up with somebody who is and make it a joint venture.

Alice's Summer Squash

Every summer, so many of the green thumbs I know report of large quantities of squash in their harvest. The peas may wither, the melon may never grow beyond golfball-size, but the squash soldiers on. And there's only so much succotash one's palate can handle. This is a tasty and easy way to enjoy the abundance.

> 6 pattypan squash (yellow flying saucer–shaped squash)
> 1 ½ cups grated cheddar cheese
> 1 teaspoon minced fresh thyme
> Salt and freshly ground black pepper

Preheat the oven to 375°F. Place 6 cups water in a large soup pot over high heat and bring to a boil. Add the squash, lower the heat to medium, and simmer until tender, 10 to 15 minutes (when pressed with a fingertip, the squash should show an indentation). Meanwhile, combine the cheese, thyme, and salt and pepper to taste in medium bowl. Remove the squash from the water, drain, and let cool slightly. Set 1 squash on a cutting board and slice the cap off the top. Scoop out the insides with a spoon and add to the cheese mixture. Repeat with remaining squash. Scoop the cheese mixture into the now-empty squash shells. Bake for 10 minutes, or until the cheese melts and the top of each squash is lightly browned.

Serves 6

QUESTIONS FOR YOUR PRODUCE MANAGER

Here are a few questions to ask when you are buying your produce:

- Where was it grown?
- When was it harvested?
- Has it been chilled or treated to prolong shelf life?
- Is it organic?
- If it's not organic, were chemical inputs used?
- If chemical inputs were used, how often and how were they applied?

PROFILE: HALL GIBSON

Every now and then we all meet someone or go through something, and the rug is pulled right out from underneath our expectations. The day I set out for Ryder Farm, in Brewster, New York, it was clear and cold, a bright winter afternoon. Not ten minutes and about five miles later, a gusting snow was swirling around my car and I had to strain to make out the driveway leading up to the farm. "That's the Yankee clipper for you," explained Hall Gibson, the farm's longtime manager, as I shook the snow from my coat and made my way into his cozy kitchen. He described the sudden weather phenomenon that we were experiencing and how it was named after the high-speed tall ships that had the ability to seemingly appear out of nowhere.

I'd come to the farm to hear Hall's views on organic farming, to find out how his CSA (Community Supported Agriculture) program works and maybe join, and to listen to some history about the centuries-old farm.

I wasn't expecting to learn about weather and ships, or many of the other things I discovered that day.

And then there was Hall himself. You could describe him as motivated, idealistic, a visionary. Or as he himself puts it, "a wool-gatherer, a cloud-nine type." Words you might use to describe a kid fresh out of college, eager to make the world a better place. Here's the thing, though: Hall Gibson is eighty-three years old, and he's worked for almost thirty years on a farm that has been in the Ryder family since 1795.

He's a dreamer. But a dreamer who manages one of the largest, most beautiful chunks of land north of New York City, "one hundred and twenty-five acres in the suburbs, a sanctuary, if you will," as he describes it. Hall married into the Ryder family, and when the farm was on the verge of being sold in 1977, he stepped in, trading the suburban life that he and his wife, Kay, and their three children had enjoyed for many years in Virginia for northeastern farm life. Before, they'd spent vacations on the property but hadn't ever considered a permanent move. But, as Hall describes it, "The idea of selling this place—the idea appalled me, so I decided to try and do something about it. My scheme was to see if I could come here and do something to keep the farm from being sold."

And that's just what he did. Today, Hall explains, "The farm with its homestead is the main cohesive influence in this far-flung family. Very few families today can gather at a two hundred-year-old homestead to bind family ties and much shared heritage." With a background in environmentalism, he decided to farm organically (the farm has been certified organic since 1985). "I think if you're an environmentalist and you don't support organic, there is something wrong with you. You're not really environmentally friendly all the way. So I was determined that when I started in '78 on my own that I'd be organic, and that's what I tried to do. But I didn't know much about it, and it was rough."

But things got a little easier every year, as the late-blooming farmer learned more and more about the land and how to coax from it some of the most delicious fruits and vegetables around. He did very well selling his produce at the Greenmarket in New York City until he stopped in 1997, when the long days at the market started to get to him, on top of the hard work of keeping the farm going. As every farmer knows, it's always something—a greenhouse roof to be replaced, hiring enough seasonal helpers, not to mention the whims of nature. "One thing I've learned since becoming a farmer . . . was that the deadlines in farming are the most real deadlines that you'll ever have. The sun doesn't stop or wait or stand still. The season moves in and things have to happen. Or else."

At that point, he'd already started a small CSA, which now has grown to include eighty members and takes most of his attention. Some of the members work on the farm, and all of them enjoy produce that has literally been just-picked, tasty, and perfectly ripe. For many of them, a trip to Ryder Farm for a weekly pickup or just a chance to visit with Hall is a matter of a few blocks. It's local, it's organic, and it's delicious.

When he's not in the field, the idealist in Hall Gibson comes out and he turns his focus to nothing short of a revolution in farming. "We've got to look into the twenty-first century and where we're going. . . . What I'm trying to do is in a sense revolutionize the way organic farming is done. From the method in the field to the equipment. Farmers now are using equipment designed and produced back fifty or sixty years ago. . . . We need modern, appropriate tractors and implements to farm in an environmentally proper way."

Hall has received grants from the USDA to perfect some alternative machinery and methods that allow him to work in partnership with the land. "What I'm trying to do is to get as close to the natural state of the soil as you can and still be farming. Because farming is an artificial thing to do. Nature doesn't farm, it doesn't grow things in rows. . . . There are ways of farming that are much more like nature and much more conserving of the environment than traditional farming methods." He calls such methods "deep organic."

He also spearheads a movement called LIFE, Local Initiatives in Food and the Environment, which aims to "bring fresh, healthful food to America's suburbs by actually growing most of that food in gardens of one acre or less within the suburbs themselves." The idea grew from his realization that food should be grown where the people are, not on thousands of acres in sparsely populated land, the way much of industrially produced food is. "Well, you can't grow much food in the inner city," he explains. "And the other extreme is out in the country where you have lots of land but not many people to buy the food, so what's in between, where most people live? Suburbs." LIFE is about taking control of food production and consumption, and of working with nature, not against it. And it just may be the solution to the powerful issue that drives Hall to do the farming he does: "Are we going to remain supine under the ever more dominating agribusiness Goliath?" If, as he'd like it, the answer is a resounding "No!" then we'd be wise to listen to the "cloud-nine types" out there such as Hall, who have the vision and experience necessary for the battle.

RYDER FARM
404 Starr Ridge Road
Brewster, New York 10509
Phone: 845-279-3984
www.ryderfarmcsa.org

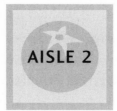

AISLE 2

THE MEAT COUNTER

My husband and I were on a road trip a couple of years back, peeling across the Midwest on motorcycle. Suddenly it hit us—an indescribable funk filled the air. It was so thick my eyes started to water. We were sending hand signals back and forth (no talking on the bike) to go faster, to get past it, but the smell just got worse as we made our way. Then we came over a hill and there it was, stretching out almost to the horizon. It looked sort of like a chessboard, except there were more black squares than not. It took a while to get close enough for our eyes to catch up to our noses—to figure out that what we were looking at was a huge sort of cow city. And the black squares? They weren't full of mud, I can tell you that.

This was my first glimpse of a commercial feedlot, and I just couldn't believe my eyes. I had heard of ILOs (Intensive Livestock Operations), but my uninformed visions of them were based on a childhood visit to my great-grandfather's family farm in South Carolina—happy cows, just more of them. These memories in no way could have come close to what lay before me. Thousands upon thousands of animals, shoulder-to-shoulder and knee-deep in their own filth. I didn't think it could be real. I half-expected someone to come into the frame and holler "cut." But it was real and it was sad, and it is a large part of why you are holding this book in your hands. I had to find out the how and why of the meat industry. Here's what I discovered about not only those cattle, but poultry and hogs as well.

INDUSTRIAL AGRICULTURE SNAPSHOT

As the *Los Angeles Times* reported, "After decades of consolidation, four companies sell more than 80% of the beef in America."[1] While vertical integration, a term used to describe how one company controls multiple aspects of the food chain, has put the majority of food production in the hands of a few, very powerful conglomerates this phenomenon is particularly resonant in meat production. There's a difference between vertical integration in terms of crops and vertical integration in terms of meat: Not many people find themselves defending the dignity of the wheat as it is harvested. In evaluating meat production, more emotional elements can and rightfully should come into play in any discussion. Such considerations are often woefully lacking in a system that is often run remotely by a CEO who never steps foot on the farm. Sonny Faison, describing his parent company, Smithfield ("the pork people"), as "the Ford Motor of livestock agriculture," says that "only the least-cost producer survives in agriculture."[2] This philosophy of efficiency and profitability drives the meat industry, which refers to animals as "production units."

Vertical integration by large conglomerates—corporate structures that give such companies control of multiple facets of the business, such as ownership of the seed, the fertilizer to grow it, the processing, packaging, and shipping units—leaves little room for small, independent players. When a company gets this tight of a grip on the market, it can easily put small farmers out of business by pricing the cost of feed, shipping, and processing out of their reach.

Farmers who are not put out of business often make do by working under contract for the larger company that dictates what they can raise, how they can raise it, and what they will be paid for it. This system locks the farmers into razor-thin profit margins that net them an increasingly lower paycheck. Ed Blair, one of the ranchers interviewed by Michael Pollan for the *New York Times*, explains, "Hell, my dad made more money on 250 head than we do on 850."[3] The volume of America's most popular meat animals—cattle, pigs, and fowl—puts them in the crosshairs of a system based entirely on economy.

Sadly, such a philosophy means that the humane treatment of animals, care of the land on which they are raised, and even human health and welfare often fall by the wayside. All of which might be less contemptible if it were for the greater good. If it were necessary to feed a starving nation or increase the nutritional value of our food supply, as the industry bigwigs would have you believe, these might be mitigating circumstances that justify the system. But it's not. It's all about the Benjamins, the bottom line of the handful of companies that designed a system that is bad for animals, the environment, our economy, and our health.

While one might argue that the modern meat industry is vastly improved since Upton Sinclair's *The Jungle* exposed the atrocities that plagued the system in the early 1900s, I would say that the problems are just different. Luckily, the industrial model isn't the only way to do things. After this brief overview of such unsavory practices, I'll introduce you to some ranchers who are reviving a sane, compassionate system for raising farm animals.

Beef

Corn-fed beef. Sounds like the heartland. Images of amber waves of grain. But the commercial grain industry, as described in Aisle 4: Grains,

Oils, and Sweeteners, is not only destructive to the environment, human health, and the economy, it is also at the epicenter of many problems that exist at the meat counter.

Corn and soy grains are a large part of the diet for most meat animals in America, yet nothing could be more unhealthy for a cow. Why? Cows are ruminants, animals that have four chambers in their stomachs that allow them to convert grass into protein. They, along with other ruminants like sheep, goats, and bison, are unique in their ability to accomplish this task. This gift makes them extremely efficient, solar-powered protein machines. A little sun, fresh water, and an assortment of grasses to munch are basically all they need to thrive.

And that's pretty much how they did get on for quite some time. They were put out to pasture, allowed to graze, and were moved around from field to field as they exhausted patches of the meadow. Tending them was a noble profession. Gauchos, cowboys, even Babe the Pig—legendary figures with the same 9 to 5—kept the animals together in a herd, moving them around as necessary. The animals got to spend their days basking in the sunshine, doing what they did best, and in return, the herder got an ample supply of complex protein. The circle of life was complete.

So what went wrong? Michael Pollan, whose writings have opened many eyes to the perils of industrial agriculture, sums up the shift in ranching that occurred just after World War II: "So because of the improvements in technology in American agriculture—but specifically because of chemical agriculture, because of chemical fertilizer—we were able to get so much corn off the land that they didn't know how to get rid of it. So the USDA made it its policy to encourage people to feed corn . . . to cows."[4] As a result, the daily ration of an American cow shifted dramatically in the 1950s to a diet that is largely grain based.

The rich, starchy corn diet causes a host of health problems in ruminants that simply aren't designed to eat this way. Daily doses of antibiotics are included in the feed to treat some of the illnesses, such as liver abscesses, caused by the unnatural diet. However, the sub-therapeutic use of the drugs is causing health concerns both on and off the farm. The systematic administration of antibiotics does not make the animal healthy. It can only prolong the animal's life for a limited time, during which it serves as a petri dish for the evolution of pathogens, as Jo Robinson writes in her book, *Why Grassfed Is Best!*[5] Additionally, Michael Pollan says, "Most of the antibiotics sold in America end up in animal feed—a practice that, it is now generally acknowledged, leads directly to the evolution of new antibiotic-resistant 'superbugs.'"[6] Some scientists believe that if the systematic administration of antibiotics in the feedlot continues, it will be harder to cure food-borne illness.

That could be a problem in a system whose design creates a fertile environment for the spread of pathogens. It all starts with the diet, which is augmented with a variety of additives to grow the animals as quickly as possible. One of the ranchers Pollan interviewed offered this comparison: "In my grandfather's day, steers were 4 or 5 years old at slaughter. . . . In the 50s . . . it was 2 or 3. Now we get there at 14 to 16 months."[7] To accomplish this goal, the cow is injected with growth hormones and fed a diet designed to increase bulk that includes corn, liquified fat, protein supplement, liquid vitamins, those antibiotics, and a bit of alfalfa hay and corn silage for roughage. The diet can also, according to FDA rules, include feather meal, pig and fish protein, and chicken manure.[8] In a measure to protect against diseases such as mad cow (Bovine Spongiform Encephalopathy, or BSE), which are transmitted when animals ingest feed containing infected tissue, the 1997 Animal Feed Rule prohibits the use of most mammalian material in ruminant feed.[9] However, there are still exceptions being taken, such as the feeding of chicken litter and restaurant scraps to cows, which can both contain bovine proteins, and the feeding of bovine blood meal to calves—practices that leave the door open to the continued spread of mad cow.

The day-to-day existence of the animal is spent eating this absurd concoction and doing not much else—less movement = low feed requirements = a cheaper feed bill. They are confined in huge outdoor pens—feedlots that can house one hundred thousand animals—until they reach a profitable weight. The thick layer of waste in the feedlot isn't just unsightly and odorous; it's dangerous. The proliferation of bacteria in the feedlot is so great that there are scientists who believe that, left unchecked, these organisms can evolve into airborne pathogens.

Evolution of barnyard pathogens is already sickening eaters. E. coli is a naturally occurring bacteria that, in a healthy animal, is not a serious threat to human health. Bacteria that have become accustomed to the alkaline environment of a healthy animal's gut cannot survive in the acid bath of the human stomach, if ingested. However, because a corn-based diet acidifies the animal's gut, making its pH more similar to that of a human's, the bacteria can leap species much more successfully—it can survive ingestion and remain strong enough to cause serious illness.[10] One such strain, E. coli 0157:H7—the bug at the center of the "Jack-in-the-Box" illnesses that sickened at least seven hundred people, hospitalized two hundred, and killed four—is relatively new.[11] "It wasn't isolated until the early 1980s—and . . . it essentially doesn't exist in the gut of animals that eat grass. It is a problem associated with feeding animals corn."[12]

Industrialized farming in general, but of beef specifically, also affects the health of the economy by making the United States more dependent on foreign oil. When you add up all of the petroleum it takes to make the fertilizers and pesticides to grow the corn, combine that with the trucking necessary to ship them to the farm, you have essentially turned the cow, an ecologically sustainable solar powered protein source, into a gas guzzler. Pollan estimates that in a steer's lifetime, it will have "consumed" roughly 284 gallons of oil.[13]

Poultry and Pork

Factory farming is not limited to beef production. Increased demand for "white meat" has brought sweeping change to the poultry and pork industries.

The cholesterol and fat fears that began to gather steam in this country in the 1970s led poultry companies like Perdue and Tyson to industrialize quickly to keep up with the soaring demands of former beef eaters who were no longer enjoying red meat.[14] (Between 1982 and 1992 turkey production doubled and broiler and chicken meat increased by nearly 70 percent.[15]) Poultry producers adopted a factory farming system that is worse than the cattle feedlots.

At least the cattle get "fresh" air and sunshine. Poultry are housed in gigantic hangars that hold tens of thousands of birds, and fecal dust fills the air. The birds are crammed so tightly into metal cages that they often resort to cannibalism out of the sheer stress of their living conditions. Commonly, a bird's beak is removed to minimize injury to its neighbors and reduce the chance of infectious wounds from nervous pecking.

The size of our poultry market is not based on the industry's need to nourish a hungry America—it is designed to feed our desire for only the "best" part of the animal, the breast. Flocks are being bred to produce more breast meat, even if the animal is not structurally suited. Poultry breasts are now so large that the birds often cannot support their own weight. Because our population favors white meat so heavily, the majority of dark meat is exported to countries such as Mexico and Russia. Perversely, only a small part of the population in these countries can afford the luxury of imported goods.

To capitalize on the demand for white meat, the pork industry has responded in kind, adopting a similar farming system and positioning pork as "The Other White Meat" by breeding the "pinkness" out of its product.[16] Hogs are also isolated in huge, sunless hangars where they are raised, as they say in the industry, "from squeal to meal." Like poultry, they are crammed into cages, and unless their tails are removed, or "docked" as it's called, they would be chewed off by their cage mates because of the stressful conditions. Their teeth are broken off so as not to injure the overburdened teats of sows forced to farrow litters engineered to bring up to twice the birth yield.[17] These animals often endure broken bones, open sores, large cancerous tumors, and a host of other ailments. Left untreated, sick or injured animals die or are made so unprofitable that they are killed, processed into meal, and fed back to their cage mates.[18]

Currently scientists are working to alter the DNA of caged animals, identifying and removing the gene that causes stress so the animal won't react adversely to its tight living quarters—essentially making the animal oblivious to its torture.

Scientific manipulation is eliminating the biodiversity of the U.S. farm animal population. Just like crops that are all planted with the same seed, homogenization leaves an entire animal population vulnerable to disease. Any vulnerability will be shared by the entire group—an Achilles' heel that, if attacked, could rapidly diminish if not destroy the entire population.

As with cattle, antibiotics are also a large part of other animals' diets, which can lead to the same kinds of human health concerns. Although the poultry industry claims to have lessened the usage of antibiotics, the pork industry has made no similar effort. Through the systematic administration of drugs, hogs are kept healthy enough to gain weight. Then the drugs are ceased a week before slaughter, in which time many animals contract pneumonia and are slaughtered in a diseased state.[19]

It's not only the farm population that suffers. The communities that surround these operations are often faced with nearly unlivable conditions because of their proximity to the farms. Factory hog farms commonly emit copious amounts of animal waste produced in their facilities into huge open-air pits called lagoons. The ammonia discharges into the air and is often blamed for the high incidence of respiratory, gastrointestinal, and infant sicknesses among people who live nearby.[20] According to Environmental Defense, one of the leading organizations for environmental activism, "Hog factories pour more nitrogen pollution (as ammonia) into the air of the coastal region than all of the municipal and industrial sources combined."[21] On occasion, lagoons burst or overflow, leaching their contents into the surrounding soil and water resources. As described on pages 95–96, run-off from chicken operations on the Eastern Seaboard is under suspicion of causing the proliferation of Pfiesteria bacteria in area water resources, killing swaths of marine life and sickening water-goers.

Slaughterhouse

The animals that survive the factory farming system—whether they are cattle, poultry, or hogs—are trucked often hundreds of miles (a number die on the way) to the slaughterhouse. The United States has the fastest, most efficient slaughterhouses in the world. Sounds good, but as Jeremy Rifkin states in his book *Beyond Beef*, rapid meat production can have negative consequences. "The drive for increased efficiency and profit has resulted in the inhumane treatment of both animals and workers, as well as increased health risks to the consumers of beef products."[22] The speed of processing—sixteen thousand hogs, for example, are killed every eight hours at Smithfield's Tar Heel plant[23]—makes inspection, which is done by sight, an unreliable tool in this environment. There are just too many animals to evaluate properly in too little time.

Animals arrive at the slaughterhouse caked in their own pathogen-ridden excrement. All are supposed to be stunned before slaughter, but there have been many reports of animals that were scalded or even skinned and eviscerated alive.[24] High-pressure hoses and cold-water baths that are supposed to remove fecal material only bury it deeper into the carcass.[25] The animals are slaughtered and butchered by a battalion of low-wage workers, who repeat the same cuts thousands of times a day. Conditions for the workers are reported to be barbaric. Charlie LeDuff, reporting for the *New York Times,* worked at a slaughterhouse in the summer of 2000 and reported that the appalling conditions led to an employee turnover rate of 100 percent annually.[26]

Machinery has been brought in to speed the process and reduce manual labor, but these mechanical methods have proved problematic as well. One of the most controversial practices, Advanced Recovery Systems, is designed to strip the small amounts of tissue that cling to the carcass of a butchered animal. In doing so, the processor can add a few more dollars to his profit margin from this otherwise unrecoverable material. However, the machine is so aggressive in its action that it pulls nerve tissue from the carcass—the ingestion of which has been linked to the transmission of mad cow disease.

Combined with consolidation and vertical integration (one company controlling multiple aspects of the food chain)—thirteen large packing-houses now slaughter most beef in America[27]—we have a recipe for disaster. As vertical integration leads to more meat being processed at fewer locations, the industry becomes increasingly susceptible to widespread food-borne illness. An outbreak at any one of these facilities has wide-reaching impact.

The Role of the United States Department of Agriculture (USDA)

American consumers are often under the assumption that the USDA seal on their meat—the blue ink stamp sometimes seen on the side of their roast or a sticker on the packaging—is proof of a government-enforced promise of clean, if not pristine, food products. This promise is not always so. While the USDA has developed procedures for inspecting, grading, and labeling meat, such systems are often compromised by human error or poorly constructed criteria, or are based on an honor system that depends entirely on the integrity of the producer.

INSPECTION

The USDA and its regulatory agency, the Food Safety and Inspection Service (FSIS), are responsible for ensuring that meat, poultry, and egg products are safe for human consumption. All meat that is sold across state lines is inspected by federal employees who are paid with your tax dollars. (Meat sold within a state must be certified by a state program that is equal in stringency to the federal guidelines.) Yet these agencies have demonstrated that when they do find health violations, they do not have the authority to affect change. The Centers for Disease Control estimates that 76 million illnesses, 325,000 hospitalizations, and 5,000 deaths are caused by food-borne pathogens annually.[28] Considering that many eaters fail to recognize symptoms of food-related illnesses, often confusing symptoms with those of the flu or believing they have a "twenty-four-hour bug," these numbers could be much higher. Evidence of the impotence of the FSIS surfaces with every new outbreak. Take the case of Nebraska Beef, Ltd., for example. As the *New York Times* reported in 2003, government agencies were powerless to shut Nebraska Beef down, even after they received multiple citations for sanitation violations.[29] Senator Richard J. Durbin (D) said, "Our scientific inspection system should be a watchdog, not a lap dog. . . . We are not doing enough to protect consumers and families."[30]

GRADING

The ubiquitous USDA shield and grading ranks, which include "Prime," "Choice," and "Select," that you may have seen posted at the meat counter, on packages in the supermarket display case, or on the menu at the steakhouse, are often interpreted by eaters as evidence of constant and vigilant government oversight. In fact, they are used largely to denote the amount of fat in a cut. They are the top three tiers of an eight-tier system that USDA inspectors use to describe the amount of marbling (white specks of fat that dot the tissue) in cuts of beef, veal, lamb, yearling mutton, and mutton, with "Prime" containing the most marbling and "Canner," the lowest of the eight grades, having the least. (Genetic streamlining of hogs has rendered pork so uniform that grading at the retail level is unnecessary.[31]) High levels of fat in beef are relatively new and are the direct result of feeding animals a rich diet of corn and keeping them confined in the feedlot. Grazing animals, like the majority of cattle raised in the United States not so long ago, are relatively lean. It wasn't until after World War II that the USDA—faced with a glut of corn—designed a system to reward and popularize the high fat content of beef raised on grain. That grading system has become synonymous with flavor and, like "corn-fed," such descriptors have come to mean a wholesome product to many consumers. Don't be fooled—these grades are not a guarantee of flavor or, necessarily, of safety.

REVIVING REAL FOOD

The current practices of the meat industry have led some people to avoid eating meat entirely. They don't want to have anything to do with this system. I can't say I blame them. If such abstinence were the only way out, I might choose it, too. But don't give up your burger or chicken pot pie just yet. There are alternatives—and they're delicious.

Buy Meat from Pastured Animals

At the furthest end of the nonindustrialized spectrum, and what some would consider the gold standard of meat, are animals raised entirely on pasture. My husband was born in Argentina where cattle are traditionally raised this way, and we made a pilgrimage there a few years ago. The reputation of Argentines as meat eaters is well documented, and I was thrilled to partake in this part of my husband's heritage. The meat was absolutely delicious, far better than the usual T-bone in the United States. I couldn't understand how the same animal could taste so different.

It wasn't until I came back from my trip and started reading about the problems with the way we in the United States raise our cattle that it started to make sense. In Argentina, much of the cattle are traditionally grazed on the pampas, the vast and beautiful open spaces that make up a great deal of the country. Unlike our cattle, many of these animals roam and munch grass all day. As a result, the composition of much of the beef in Argentina—as it is in any grass-fed animal—is hugely different than that of a factory-farmed, corn-fed beast.

Pasturing animals isn't just for cattle. Often a variety of animals graze over the same meadows in a carefully calibrated dance that is mutually beneficial to the animals and the fields. One of the most renowned proponents of grass-fed farming, Joel Salatin, runs his Polyface Farm in Virginia this way: "Chickens sanitize the pasture behind the cows by debugging. Cows graze, harvesting their own forage, rather than us me-chanically harvesting it for them. Pigs turn compost. Rabbits mow under the orchard."[32]

Ranching in this manner has numerous advantages to land, beast, and eater. If careful attention is paid to the condition of the pasture (some of these farmers call themselves "grass farmers" because they depend on its growth so exclusively), no man-made inputs like fertilizers or pesticides are required. And, because animals graze over large areas of land, their waste breaks down naturally over time without having a negative impact on the pasture or their community.

Allowing animals to eat the diet they were evolved to graze, peck, or root as their instinct drives them has myriad benefits to the animals' well-being. Their natural behavior and exposure to fresh air and sunshine keeps their stress level low, so they are less susceptible to stress-related illnesses and don't exhibit aggressive behavior that causes them to snap and bite at each other or themselves. Pasture-raised animals do not require large doses of antibiotics to survive their feed, so they won't be passing such drugs on to you or contributing to the proliferation of drug-resistant bac-teria. Eating grass maintains a properly alkaline pH level in the stomach of cattle, which—because human stomachs have an acidic pH—is a natural check and balance system that prevents us from getting seriously ill from any pathogens, such as E. coli, that we might ingest. Additionally, an ani-mal that eats only grass, or a combination of grass and organic feed, is not susceptible to mad cow and other diseases that are contracted by eating feed that contains animal protein.

The meat from such animals—and, as discussed in Aisle 5: Dairy, the milk and eggs they provide—is growing in popularity as a superior dining choice. According to writer Michael Pollan, "A growing body of research suggests that many of the health problems associated with eating beef are really problems with [eating] corn-fed beef."[33] In her book *Why Grassfed Is Best!* Jo Robinson explains that not only is the amount of fat in grass-fed meats lower than that of grain-fed animals (she contends that grass-fed beef has the fat equivalent of skinless chicken breasts), but the type of fat found in grass-fed meat is beneficial to human health. Pasture-raised meats contain high levels of omega-3 fatty acids, acids that are essential to normal human growth and development. Diets rich in omega-3s have been linked to lower incidence of cardiovascular problems, depression, brain disorders such as attention deficit disorder and dementia, and invasive breast cancer. Pasture-raised animals also have higher levels of beta carotene and CLA (conjugated linoleic acid, a compound that is being studied for its muscle-building properties and has been linked to reduced risk of cancer).[34]

And, all science aside, pastures are simply more beautiful than hundreds of square miles of animal hangars and waste lagoons. Among those lush, green fields it would not be unlikely to spot heritage breed animals. Such animals maintain highly desirable traits such as superior mothering skills, strong immune systems, and truer flavor that have been lost in the over-bred factory species but make heritage breeds well-suited to the open-air lifestyle. Heritage breeds are also carefully mated to maintain their genetic diversity, an important aspect of sustainability and hardiness. (See the Profile on Cabbage Hill Farm on page 85 for more about heritage breeds.)

Meat from animals that are raised entirely on pasture and from heritage breeds can taste strikingly different from that which you might find wrapped in plastic at the area MegaMart. The meat, whether it's beef, lamb, chicken, or pork, is not bloated with toxins and additives, so it's "truer"—some might say stronger. Peter Hoffman, the chef at Savoy restaurant in New York City, says that the pork raised by Flying Pigs Farm in Shushan, New York, is "astonishing in its rich flavor."[35] After having tasted it, some eaters liken dining on factory-farmed chicken to eating tofu. Like wine connoisseurs who talk about the terroir of a vintage—the quality added by the soil whence it came—there are steak lovers among us who appreciate that these animals are raised in fresh air and sunshine and believe that the flavor of dinner reflects all that this entails.

Buy meat from animals that have been raised in the open air, not in a feedlot or confined cage system. There is no nationally enforced standard for labeling of grass-fed products, so it is important to know and trust the farm from which you are buying. Such products fall into two categories:

100 PERCENT GRASS-FINISHED

Animals that fall under this heading are raised entirely on pasture. Large animals, such as cattle, that are wintered over to reach maturity are fed on stored grass and hay.

GRASS-FED

While 100 percent grass-finished meat is the ideal, more frequently ranchers are turning to a blend of diet that combines the grazing lifestyle with some supplemental grain feeding to add more flexibility to their operation. A number of these ranchers contend that even though all meat was raised almost entirely on pasture before the introduction of feedlots and it all tasted this way, eaters' palates have changed and they prefer a less assertive flavor in their protein choices. And it is true that some eaters prefer a milder flavor. To mellow the taste of the meat, animals are taken off of the field for a period of time before slaughter to increase their intramuscular fat content and bring their flavor more in line with commercially raised products. Other ranchers supplement their pastured animals' diets with grain to produce more predictable results—the flavor of the meat doesn't shift with the seasonality of the grasses. And some "winter" their animals on a blend of grain and forage until the salad bar of spring grass returns.

While any increase in time on pasture is admirable and benefits the environment, the eater, and the animal, it should be noted that these benefits begin to decline as soon as an animal is taken off of a grass-based diet. Finishing an animal on grain before slaughter makes the meat higher in saturated fat and lower in CLA and omega-3s.[36]

Grass-Fed Veal Burgers with Chipotle Peppers

I've never been much of a veal eater. But when I came across a great deal on ground veal on one of the Internet sites from which I buy grass-fed meat, I bought a pound and experimented. I came up with this recipe, which has quickly become a family favorite. These burgers are a nice change from traditional beef burgers—the flavor of the meat is more subtle and makes a good foil for the smoky peppers. And they are terrific with extra-sharp provolone cheese melted on top.

1 pound grass-fed ground veal
1½ teaspoons garlic powder
1 tablespoon olive oil
1½ teaspoons dried parsley
¼ cup finely chopped fresh cilantro
2 teaspoons salt
1 tablespoon dried chipotle pepper flakes

Lightly mix all the ingredients together in a large bowl. Form into 4 patties and grill or fry over medium-high heat for 3 minutes, then flip and cook 5 to 7 minutes more.

Serves 4

Buy Directly from the Farmer

VISIT A FARM

Finding pastured meat can be a challenge. Your best bet is to buy directly from the farmer. If you can find one close by, I encourage you to pay them a visit. Your time will be richly rewarded. I found a great purveyor, Meadow Raised Meats, a cooperative of like-minded ranchers. One bite of their sirloin and my husband swooned; it took him right back to the pampas of Argentina. To get a firsthand look at a grass-fed operation, I drove out to one of the Meadow Raised Meats farms, Skate Creek in East Meredith, New York, at the beginning of spring—or at least that was the season on my calendar. It's quite a way from my house in Connecticut, but it looked like I had driven all the way to December. Everything was covered in ice. I felt like I was driving through a glass forest. But Amy Kenyon and Craig Haney, who owned and operated the farm together at the time, warmed me up with a cup of hot tea and gave me the tour. Their sunny slopes were positioned just right to catch the early thaw and we slushed through mud to meet the animals. Amy and Craig knew each animal, and had stories for most. I thought it might be a bit off-putting to look into the eyes of the animals. But it wasn't like that at all and, from what I've read, most people who visit a pasture-raised animal farm have a similar feeling.

There's a level of comfort knowing that these animals are so well cared for. Craig used a word, "reverence," that I think really hit it on the head. I felt that in some way my participation in the process—by choosing this type of meat—made it less barbaric, that by playing a part I was accepting my place in the animal kingdom. I wasn't just a rat waiting for my pellet to come out of the chute; I was an active participant in the food chain, making a decision that, while shortening the life of this animal, did not cause it to suffer or struggle through a painful and confusing existence. We talked about it a little. Amy said that someone once asked her how she could eat an animal that she had raised from birth and Amy replied, "How can you go out to dinner and eat something with absolutely no idea where it came from?" (See the Profile on Stafford Enterprises on page 82 for more information about humane practices.)

INTERNET/MAIL ORDER

If you haven't a farm nearby, use mail order to bring one to your doorstep. Generally, I am not in favor of shipping food great distances. But for some products, particularly those such as pastured meats that are not readily available in the marketplace, such purchasing methods support sustainable operations until their popularity reaches the critical mass necessary to be stocked with regularity at many retail outlets.

FINDING A RANCHER

Whether it's on the farm, through a Web site, or an 800 number, I appreciate the direct communication I have with the rancher. I can explore the nuances of their practices and feel confident about what I'm putting on my dinner plate. Here's how to make contact with a rancher in your area:

www.eatwellguide.org
A directory of resources for sustainably raised animal products.

www.eatwild.com
A national directory of producers of grass-fed meats from Jo Robinson, author of *Why Grassfed Is Best!*

STOCK UP

For the most part pastured animals are slaughtered seasonally, so if you want fresh meat, you need to sing the same "eat seasonal" chant that holds true in every corner of the market and cook up fresh cuts as they become available, or freeze them. Many ranchers will sell their meat in quarters or sides for an averaged price per pound. The animal is "broken-down" and wrapped into meal-sized portions, ready for your freezer. Hook up with a friend or two and split the order if you don't have the storage space or the budget for a lot of product.

If You Can't Buy Directly, Buy Indirectly

If you would like to sample some nonindustrialized meat, these alternatives are a great place to start. Co-ops and natural food stores often stock grass-fed, organic, and exotic meats. If they don't have what you are interested in, they might be able to order it, so don't be afraid to ask. Although it is not an item that they have in stock, my local natural food store hooks me up with ducks that are raised humanely on a regular basis. All they ask is a little advance notice—about a week—and they are happy to oblige.

Find a Butcher

Not so long ago, every town had its own butcher. I had one when I lived in New York City, and it changed the way I looked at my dinner plate. I never knew my menu for the evening until I walked through the door and got the answer to "What's good today?" Nick, the owner, would fill me in and tell me the story of my food. Where it came from and what I should do with it. He taught me which cuts to braise and which to sear—he even took the mystery out of how to cook a proper steak.

But butchers do much more than provide delicious cooking tips. They act as your advocate in the marketplace. They have longstanding relationships with the farmers, producers, and wholesalers whose goods they represent, so they can provide you with a rich history of the items you're selecting. They also provide an additional safety check. Freshness is not a black-and-white issue; there are degrees to it. I don't want to be too far into the gray when I'm buying my food. I want to know "how" fresh—"just in this morning" is a far cry from "won't make you too sick." Only a knowledgeable purveyor—who knows when the food was caught, cured, or aged—can give me the level of information that I'm looking for.

Butchers can also vet out superior quality. Good food has nuance and character, faults and attributes like any entity of distinction. Skilled purveyors are trained to appreciate, evaluate, and translate these subtle differences. They don't need a USDA stamp to distinguish a flavorful cut of meat from one that will cook up like shoe leather—they can tell by looking at it. Such shop owners can also special-order things for you. The holiday roast that is the perfect size to feed your crowd. The ten pounds of veal bones you need to try your hand at demi-glace.

Nick's Steak

This is the recipe handed down to me from my butcher, Nick. It's simple and turns out foolproof medium steaks every time. It absolutely requires a good skillet—cast iron would be ideal. An exhaust hood or open window is handy—this is a smoky one.

> 1 tablespoon kosher salt
> Two 1½-inch-thick steaks, preferably bone-in

Place a large skillet over the highest flame for 5 minutes to preheat. Be careful, as the pan will become ferociously hot. Sprinkle half of the salt in the pan and carefully lay the steaks on top of the salt. The steaks will sear and pop with great commotion. Do not move them. The steaks will release from the bottom of the pan when browned, after 5 to 7 minutes. Remove the steaks to a plate, sprinkle the remaining salt in the pan, and return the steaks, uncooked-side-down, to the pan and cook until they release from the pan, about another 5 to 7 minutes, or until internal temperature reaches 145°F for medium rare. (Insert thermometer through side of steak to obtain an accurate reading.) Remove the steaks to a clean plate and allow to rest 5 minutes before serving.

Serves 2

Know Your Labels

Following are the USDA definitions of some words that you may find at the meat counter. Their meanings probably vary greatly from what you might expect or would find in your Webster's Dictionary.

ORGANIC

As it applies to meat, the National Organic Standards stipulate that:

- The animals are given no antibiotics or growth hormones.
- The animals are fed an organic diet.
- They are not fed animal by-products.
- They may not be bio-engineered.
- Organic meat cannot be treated with ionizing radiation.

All of these criteria must be meticulously documented by the farmer and verified on site by a government certified inspector. Only then can products be labeled "organic" and carry the USDA Organic seal.

An organic label does not address all of the troubling issues we face in the current food production model. For example, animals that are fed an organic diet may still be on a grain-based regimen that is unnatural for their systems, although that feed will be organic. However, organic meats do offer some clear advantages to their industrialized counterparts:

- Because organic meats are guaranteed to be hormone- and antibiotic-free, they will not be passing these residues on to you.
- While the stipulations on animal care are not clearly outlined in the standards, it would be difficult to raise such an animal in substandard facilities because they cannot be dosed with antibiotics.
- The animals' organic diet ensures that they will also not be passing feed-based pesticide residue on to you.
- Because organic feed cannot contain GMOs, you are reducing the market for genetically modified commodity crops such as corn and soy.
- Until there is mandatory labeling of GMOs, the organic label is the only guarantee that you are eating a GMO-free product. (There is no production of GMO animals for human consumption at this time, but producers, particularly salmon farmers, are lobbying for the FDA to allow it.)

- Their diets cannot contain animal by-products, which are the critical vector for the transmission of diseases such as mad cow.
- The meat is not irradiated. (See page 65 for more information on irradiated meat.)

HORMONE-FREE

"Hormone-free" means raised without the use of hormones. In the United States, this term is only relevant when used on beef and lamb products. The producer must submit documentation stating that its animals received no hormones, but facilities are not inspected to validate these claims. And since all animals produce some level of hormone naturally, there is no test that can be used to screen out hormones delivered by injection.[37]

Hormones are never allowed in the raising of hogs or fowl. The label is sometimes used on pork and poultry products to lead buyers to believe that they are buying a superior product, but it in itself is completely irrelevant when used in this manner and must be followed by a statement that says, in effect, *"Federal regulations prohibit the use of hormones in poultry."*

NO ANTIBIOTICS

This phrase means that the animals—chickens, turkeys, cattle, and pigs—were never administered antibiotics. Like "hormone-free," this claim relies on the honesty of the producer. They must submit documentation to support their claim, but their facilities are not inspected. Upon arrival at the slaughterhouse, a random sampling may be taken from the flock or herd, but a negative result is not an indication that the animal was raised drug-free. Because antibiotics leave an animal's system over time, a test can only determine that there are no antibiotics present at the time of slaughter.[38]

FRESH

Ever unwrap some poultry that you just brought home from the market to find that it's hard as a rock even though it's labeled "fresh"? This happened to me one Thanksgiving. I had ordered a fresh turkey from the local supermarket for the big feast. I thought that "fresh" would actually mean never frozen. In fact, I was handed a tom that was a bird-shaped ice cube. I wasn't too happy with my turkey-sicle and was a bit panicked at the prospect of having to defrost an eighteen-pound bird overnight and get it on the table hot and ready by the next afternoon. I asked to see the manager, who said these exact words to me: "It ain't froze. It's only twenty-six degrees Fahrenheit. It's just chilled." In all my years of waiting for snow days, I thought that 32 was the magic number here.

The next day I logged on to the USDA Web site (you can do this, too; it's www.usda.gov) and discovered this: According to the USDA, poultry can be called "fresh" as long as its internal temperature does not go below twenty-six degrees. An internal temp between zero and twenty-six degrees rates a "hard-chilled" or "previously hard-chilled" description. A bird is not officially frozen until the mercury dips to below zero degrees Fahrenheit. OK, I'll tell that to Jack Frost.

FREE-RANGE

I usually see the term "free-range" when I am shopping for poultry or eggs. It makes me think of the most wholesome of farm scenes. A young girl, apron brimming with feed, sings a country ditty as she broadcasts dinner to her eager flock. Wings flapping, they scurry from all corners of the barnyard to have their meal. And for a small group of farmers, that's pretty much what they mean when they use the term "free-range" or "free-ranging." They allow their birds to scratch around outside in the fresh air and sunshine as much as their climate and the weather allow. Unfortunately, the technical definition of the term leaves a lot of room for interpretation.

According to the FDA, "free-range" or "free-roaming" products are derived from animals that have "been allowed access to the outside." This doesn't mean that the animals have actually been outside. This is how it works. You take a shed roughly the size of an airplane hangar. Fill it full of birds that stand wing to wing. At one end of the hangar, install a garage door and leave it open. The birds won't move. Their instinct to travel in a flock binds them together so tightly that they will never leave the hangar. As a matter of fact, the birds are packed together so snugly that if you put a dime under one when you introduced it to its new hangar home, you could come back at slaughter time and find that dime under the same bird.

NATURAL

The term "natural" applies only to the handling of meat and meat products from any animal after slaughter. It indicates that no artificial ingredients or colors were added to the meat and that it was not altered to change its fundamental makeup. It does not mean that the animal was raised in any specific way—it could have been fed anything up until the day it met its maker.

The USDA requires documentation from the producer on meat that bears a "Natural" label but, unlike meats labeled "Organic," there is no inspection protocol in place to verify its validity.[39]

NOT YET IN SERVICE—COUNTRY OF ORIGIN LABELING

According to the 2002 Farm Bill, the USDA is required to establish standards for mandatory country of origin labeling in 2006. Yet there is so much argument against such a requirement from the food industry, there is talk of repealing the measure. Retailers, who would be required to document the lineage of many products, say such documentation would bury them in paperwork. Producers that handle meats from multiple countries will have to find new production methods to keep the products from mingling. Government regulators fear agitating trading partners. The only group that seems to be all for it are the consumers.

The labels will not only inform eaters about the history of their dinner but also add a level of traceability for contaminated products. After the May 2003 discovery of mad cow disease in Canada, the United States immediately ceased importing beef from Canada, but it did not pull it from the shelves. This was perhaps because in the current, label-free system, such a recall would have been impossible to implement (ground meat, in particular, is a combination of domestic and imported meats, limiting the viability of tracing products back to their source). If the meat had been labeled sufficiently in the first place, it could have facilitated such a recall or, at the least, consumers could choose whether or not to buy the Canadian burger. Clear labeling puts product choice in the hands of the eater. It allows eaters to boycott products from countries with production, labor, or sanitation standards that they find sub-par.

Avoid Irradiated Meat

This term is defined by the Food Safety and Inspection Service as "the use of ionizing radiation for treating refrigerated or frozen uncooked meat, meat by-products, and certain other meat food products to reduce levels of food-borne pathogens and to extend shelf life."[40] Fruits, vegetables, spices, and grains can also be irradiated. The process exposes the food product to one of three kinds of rays (gamma, e-rays, or X-rays) in an insulated tube for a predetermined amount of time. Irradiated meat products must be labeled with either "Irradiated" in the product name or a statement such as "Treated with Radiation" or, synonymously, "Treated by Irradiation," and the label must bear the radura symbol, below, on the packaging.

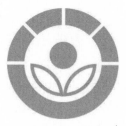

The U.S. government and the food industry support the use of irradiation as a valid method of controlling pathogens in the food supply, despite the following:

- It gives consumers a false sense of security. While irradiation reduces the levels of pathogens such as E. coli, it does not eliminate them and it provides no protection against contamination from diseases such as mad cow.
- The health impact of irradiation is not entirely known. It has been linked to cancer in some lab tests and more tests are still required to understand the full impact of the process.[41]
- It degrades the quality of the meat.[42]
- The process often results in nuclear waste.
- The equipment used to irradiate meat is expensive and will eliminate even more small farmers from the marketplace who cannot compete with conglomerates that can afford such machinery.

As was discussed in the beginning of this chapter, bacteria in meat is a byproduct of a system that prides itself on speed, efficiency, and capital gain, not quality. If the system were overhauled, such bacteria—which the meat industry claims necessitates irradiation—would not exist in the first place. Irradiation would not be necessary if meat were processed more slowly or if animals were fed a diet that was not so heavily grain based. Instead of implementing systems to sanitize contaminated meat, the meat industry should be working at the source of the problem to eliminate contamination in the first place.

Avoid "White" Veal

The pale white color of industrially raised veal is caused by penning the animal and feeding it a restricted diet that makes it anemic. The meat from a healthy young cow that is raised under more humane conditions is pink and is sometimes referred to as "baby beef."

Buy Less Luxurious Cuts of Meat

If you find that grass-fed or organic meat is adding to your grocery bill more than you'd like, try buying less expensive cuts. Instead of selecting a conventional premium cut of meat like a filet mignon, New York strip, or center-cut pork chops, buy an organic or grass-fed, but less pricey selection, such as a skirt steak, chuck roast, or pork shoulder. You'll be saving money and utilizing more of the animal, an important value of sustainability shared by a growing contingent of chefs who are building "market menus" around the cuts they are offered.

Braised Pork Shoulder with Lime

This recipe is perfect for a grass-fed cut like this pork shoulder. It uses moist cooking to enhance the juiciness of the meat and a long, slow cooking time to ensure tenderness. The lime juice further tenderizes the meat and adds an unusual flavor. It's also terrific cooked all day in a crockpot.

Juice of 8 limes (about 1 cup)
4 garlic cloves, minced
2 tablespoons coarse salt, plus more to taste
2 tablespoons dried oregano
1 tablespoon dried parsley
2 tablespoons ground cumin
1 tablespoon red pepper flakes
One 8-pound bone-in pork shoulder
3 cups water
6 tablespoons red wine vinegar

Preheat oven to 375°F. Combine ¼ cup of the lime juice, the garlic, salt, oregano, parsley, cumin, and red pepper flakes in a small bowl. Place the pork in a large roasting pan and make 1-inch long by ¾-inch deep cuts 2 inches apart all over the pork. Push about 1 teaspoon of the lime juice mixture into each incision. Pour the remaining lime juice over the pork. Roast, uncovered, until the juice is almost completely evaporated, about 30 minutes. Pour the water and vinegar over the pork, cover tightly with foil, and continue to roast for 2 hours, basting with juices halfway through. Remove the foil, sprinkle with salt to taste, and roast for another 1½ hours, basting every 20 minutes.

Remove from the oven and let the pork rest for 20 minutes, then slice into ¼-inch-thick slices. Reserve the pan juices, skim off the fat, and pass in a gravy boat at the table. Serve warm or at room temperature.

Serves 8

Have Your Hamburger Ground for You

Hamburger that is sold pre-ground often contains the meat of multiple animals. If it was packaged at the processing plant, the product can even come from thousands of carcasses, which broadens the scope of any food-borne illness considerably. To lessen your chance of contracting a food-borne illness and to control the contents of your burger, have the folks at the meat counter grind your chopped meat from a cut, such as a whole chuck roast, that you select yourself. You can even have this done at the MegaMart—just ask the folks behind the meat counter.

Eat Exotic Meats

Although some efforts have been made to subject bison to factory farming methods, they and other "wilder" meat breeds such as ostrich, goat, emu, elk, and deer offer you a much better chance at avoiding industrialized meat. The relatively small size of their population hasn't made them candidates for a system that thrives on mass production. Their lack of domestication means that they just can't tolerate the conditions; buffalo have been known to destroy even the sturdiest pens to escape.

I found buffalo at my area MegaMart. It is widely available at supermarkets like Wild Oats and Fresh Fields. You can also find ranchers online or in books such as Jo Robinson's *Why Grassfed Is Best!* (www.eatwild.com).

It Shouldn't All Taste Like Chicken— Eat a Variety of Meats

Eating a variety of meats—chicken, pork, beef, seafood, exotic meats— evens out consumer demand and takes the pressure off any single category to constantly increase production.

Don't Buy Meat That Is Veiled Behind Coatings, Colorings, or Flavorings

Uncooked, pre-marinated meat and fully cooked seasoned meats are the latest wave of innovation by the meat industry. They are industry tools for charging a high price for water and other additives. On a recent trip to the MegaMart, I looked at the fine print on a Perdue Ovenable (seasoned boneless skinless chicken breasts in an ovenproof tray), which read that the chicken contained up to 15 percent of a seasoning solution. Tyson's precooked pork tenderloin contained a whopping 20 percent of fluid. Beyond the obvious advantage of selling water at meat market prices, portion-controlling and further processing meats means that, as Jack Dunn, senior vice president for refrigerated processed meats at Tyson Foods says, "Your product is not tied as directly to a commodity market, and you're going to smooth out your earnings and you're also going to increase your returns."[43]

These products are promoted by the manufacturers as time-saving shortcuts that will give the busy family the opportunity to gather around the table and share a meal without visiting the local drive-thru.[44] It's hard to debate that. You could argue that the absence of family dining is the root of many evils and therefore any tool that allows us to break bread together is a valid one. But feeding a family isn't just about fueling up; it's about nurturing each other with nutrition, cultural tradition, and social connection. On that level, these meals fall flat. There's a reason that the Sunday roast is cooked on the weekend. Part of the enjoyment of that feast is the slow braise that fills the house with earthy aromas, enticing everyone to table. And yes, a roast takes a large part of the day to cook, but most of the time that the food cooks is unsupervised—the perfect window to grab the gang for a round of touch football or even some armchair game watching.

Or will the Sunday roast become obsolete? Let's roll forward a generation or two. If we are to believe that the only way the modern family can manage to enjoy a traditional meal like a slow-roasted pot roast is by picking up a vacu-sealed model from the chill case, then we are going to have to deal with the fact that there will be no "just like Mom used to make" memories, no Granny's secret meatloaf recipe and eventually, what? Microwaved turkey loaf on white bread for Thanksgiving?

Do your part to protect this endangered species—the home-cooked meal. Get out there and buy yourself a (hopefully, organic or grass-fed) roast, toss it in the pot, and enjoy a Sunday with your family or friends. Cook two while you are at it, and you can have that real homemade flavor all week long.

Sunday Ham Dinner

I've never been a big fan of ham covered in pineapple slices, but I do like the combination of the salty pork flavor and the sweetness of fruit. This dish uses dried fruit instead of fresh, and the result is unusual, and gorgeous to behold.

    1 cooked bone-in smoked ham, about 10 pounds
    20 whole cloves
    ⅓ cup Dijon mustard
    ½ cup apple cider vinegar
    1 cup apple juice
    2 cups sweet red wine
    1 cup pitted whole dried dates
    1 cup dried figs
    1 cup pitted dried prunes
    1 cup raisins

Preheat the oven to 350°F. Remove the skin from the ham and trim the fat to a layer about ¼-inch thick. Score the fat in a diamond pattern, and insert cloves all over. Pat the mustard over the ham and place it in a large roasting pan. Pour the apple cider vinegar and the apple juice over the ham. Bake for 1½ hours, then add the wine and dried fruit to the pan and bake another 30 minutes. Serve the ham on a large platter surrounded by the fruit.

Serves 6

Don't Pay for Water

Four dollars and ninety-nine cents per pound sounds like a high price to pay for water, but if you are buying meat, pork, or poultry that is industrially processed (from a company like Perdue or Tyson, for instance), that's exactly what you may be doing. If you read the fine print on your chicken packaging, you will often see a disclaimer along the lines of: "up to X% water retained from chilling process." According to the USDA, that percentage can be up to 8 percent. That water is big business for companies like Tyson, where in 1994 such an inclusion was calculated to add "about $40 million in annual gross profits" to their bottom line.[48]

Where does all that water come from? For the birds, it is absorbed by the carcasses when they are dunked in the chill tank at the slaughterhouse. Detractors call this cold bath "fecal soup," and say it is to blame for a large part of the contamination of our poultry supply with bacteria such as salmonella. The bloating and contamination risk could easily be eliminated by wrapping the birds in plastic before submerging them, but again, profit wins this argument for factory farmers.

But you don't have to pay for it and you certainly shouldn't have to eat it. Buy birds that have little or no added or retained water—they are sometimes marked "air chilled."

Beware Case-Ready Meat

Not long ago, beef was shipped to market in sides and quarters, birds arrived whole, and the resident butcher took it from there. Now most meat arrives boxed in small pieces to be trimmed, weighed, and packaged onsite by cutters. Some "grocers" are reducing human involvement at the store level even further by carrying "case-ready meat." Such products arrive already cut, packaged, labeled, and ready for display, like so many piles of socks. Case-ready meat has obviated the need to have a trained butcher or meat handler on staff who can vouch for the meat's safe handling and maybe even offer some advice on the best way to prepare it.

Case-ready is not in itself a sign of a bad product, but it should raise a red flag for you to investigate before you buy. To make it easier to stock, case-ready meat has often been altered to extend its shelf life. It may have had a substantial amount of water added to it in processing, been injected with significant amounts of saline solution or other preservatives, or had its packaging flushed with inert gas.[45]

In an interview at Stafford Enterprises, I spoke with Allen Williams, cofounder of the Jacob Alliance, a livestock industry consultancy, who described it best. He said, "When you buy a case-ready product . . . the consumer is buying 12 to 15 percent water. They're injecting all of their beef products with water, plus adding rosemary in there to add a little tint of flavor and to help improve tenderness. What is happening is that [Mega-Marts], because they want to be the low-cost leader, the only way to get low costs is to have the lowest quality beef product in their store that they can possibly have. . . . The big packers love [such stores] because they essentially are able to dump all their lowest quality beef products onto the

Brazilian-Style Black Beans

I got this recipe from a cook who spent a year in Brazil. The amount of garlic may look shocking, but it mellows in the cooking. The beans are meant to be a side dish, but they are so creamy that they also stand in as a hearty sauce when paired with grilled or roasted meats or fish.

¼ cup olive oil
1 small onion, finely diced
1 head garlic, cloves peeled and finely minced (see Note)
Slow-Cooked Black Beans (recipe follows)

1 teaspoon dried thyme
Salt and freshly ground black pepper

Heat the oil in a medium saucepan over medium heat. Add onion and sauté until translucent, 5 to 7 minutes. Add the garlic and sauté 1 to 2 minutes, until fragrant but not brown. Add the beans and thyme, bring to a simmer, then reduce the heat to low. Cook gently, stirring occasionally, until the beans begin to lose their shape and the garlic has lost its bite, 35 to 45 minutes. Add salt and pepper to taste. Serve immediately or freeze in serving-size portions for later use.

Serves 6 to 8

NOTE: When dealing with such a large amount of garlic, it can pay to break out a helpful tool, the hand blender. Peel the cloves, place them into the 2-cup measure that came with the mixer or a small bowl, add ¼ cup olive oil, and puree to a paste. If using this method in this recipe, use only 2 tablespoons olive oil to sauté the onions and add the pureed garlic and oil mixture in place of the minced cloves.

Slow-Cooked Beans

Slow-cooked beans are a kitchen staple in my house—I always have some portions stowed in the freezer. You can use this recipe for whatever type of bean you have on hand. White beans combine with greens for an easy dinner of *Greens and Beans on Toast* (see page 206 for recipe). Black beans, made rich and smoky with the addition of a dried chile rather than the traditional ham hock, can be cooked further for the rich Brazilian-style beans described above or simply mixed in with rice for a complete dinner.

1 pound dried black or white beans
1 onion, cut in half
1 head garlic, cloves separated and peeled
1 bouquet garni (1 bay leaf, 1 teaspoon thyme, and 6 peppercorns, tied into a cheesecloth knot or placed in a tea ball)
1 dried chile, such as chipotle or ancho, if cooking black beans

Soak the beans overnight in a bowl with cold water to cover by 2 inches in the refrigerator. Strain the beans, then rinse and pick over them to remove any odd stones or deformed beans. Place the beans and the remaining ingredients in a large saucepan and add enough water to cover by 2 inches. Place over high heat and bring to a boil. Reduce the heat immediately to a simmer and cook, uncovered, 1 to 2 hours (time varies greatly depending on the freshness of the beans), until the beans are just tender.

Remove the onion, garlic, bouquet garni, and dried chile, if using. Serve as a side dish or use in any recipe that calls for beans. Or cool completely, divide into freezer bags with some of the cooking liquid in each bag, and freeze for later use. This recipe can be doubled easily.

Yields approximately one quart of cooked beans

[stores]. And so beyond not getting a choice of what you want, just having to take whatever's packaged there . . . you're buying 12 to 15 percent water. In my mind that's a consumer rip-off. Not a lot of consumers are aware of that. If you take [such a] product, turn it over and . . . it'll actually have an ingredient list. That's not beef, that's sausage! You've got a

totally different product here if you have to have an ingredient list." (See the Profile on Stafford Enterprises on page 82.)

As companies such as Wal-Mart, which has sold only case-ready meat

Marinara Sauce

If you are used to getting your tomato sauce out of a can, this might be just the quick and easy recipe to convert you to homemade. It really takes no time at all and the result is tasty and fresh.

    2 tablespoons olive oil
    1 small yellow onion, finely diced
    2 garlic cloves, minced
    Pinch of dried red pepper flakes (optional)
    One 28-ounce can whole peeled tomatoes, crushed by hand
    Pinch of sugar
    Salt and freshly ground black pepper
    ¼ cup basil leaves torn into quarters (optional)

Heat the oil in a medium heavy-bottomed skillet over medium heat. Add the onion and sauté until translucent, 5 to 7 minutes. Add the garlic and red pepper flakes, if using, and sauté 1 minute, until fragrant. Add the tomatoes and stir. Reduce the heat to medium-low. Small bubbles should be appearing all over the surface of the mixture, but not splattering your stove. If speckles of sauce are sputtering out onto your stovetop, reduce the heat to low. (If you are serving with pasta, now is a good time to get your water boiling.) Continue simmering until thickened, about 20 minutes. Do not stir, or this will hamper the thickening process. Remove from the heat and add the sugar, salt and pepper to taste, and the basil, if using.

Serves 4 over pasta

since 2001, further expand into the grocery business, this practice will become ubiquitous, eliminating meat cutters at the store level and flooding shelves with preserved meat products. Stop the infiltration of such products into the food chain and enjoy fresh cuts by always supporting a manned meat counter.

Try Some Exotic Cuisines

Much of the world's population dines on satisfying dishes that use a small amount of meat just for flavoring. In this way they stretch their supply and save some money. Try it out and see if these dishes don't satisfy. Pad thai, rice and beans, and bean stew are some such dishes

Eat a Meatless Meal Once in a While

You don't have to become a vegetarian to enjoy an all-vegetable meal every now and then. Such a step, however small, does indeed take some of the pressure off the meat industry to produce at such an intense level. Throw a curve once or twice a week and serve up a meatless meal. Some good options: mushroom risotto, pasta with marinara sauce, falafel, mac and cheese, pizza, or just a nice big salad.

A Note About Boutique Beef

I have been hearing a lot lately about what is being referred to as "Boutique Beef," high-end products that are advertised as a more flavorful alternative to what you might find at the supermarket. They include everything from mail-order products such as Omaha Steaks to imported selections like Kobe beef, an extremely prized and expensive Japanese product, to quality domestic cuts that are "well aged." I was curious about the practices involved in raising these animals and found out they are all over the map.

The Omaha Steaks line, for instance, is industrialized beef that fulfills criteria the company has established for appearance and flavor. It is corn-fed, can be either prime or choice, and is generally aged for about three weeks.[46]

Some companies, such as Niman Ranch, fall in the gray area between the industrial model and a more sustainable structure. They do not administer sub-therapeutic antibiotics to any of their animals (only sick cattle are medicated) or hormones to their cattle or sheep (administration of hormones to pigs is illegal). Their animals are not fed animal by-products such as rendered protein or chicken feathers, and spend more time with their mothers and in pasture than those destined for the commodity market. Their animals, however, are "finished" on grain (they are fed grain-based diets for a period before slaughter), which some argue negates many of the benefits of grass-feeding.

"Kobe" beef is rumored to come from Japanese steers that are fed beer and massaged with sake. In Japan that may be true. In the United States, however, Kobe beef can only be guaranteed to mean one thing—that the animal gets at least some of its genes from Wagyu cattle. Whether the animal was buffed and polished or fed a diet of bonbons is up to the rancher, but it isn't certified in this country.

Another confusing "breed branding" label you might see is Certified Angus Beef. It is a marketing tool of the American Angus Association that is used to raise demand for its members' products. Beef that bears this label must be 51 percent Angus bred and meet the association's parameters of quality, but it does not signify a protocol for raising or feeding the animals in a particular manner.

Aging improves the flavor and texture of any meat by reducing its water content and allowing natural enzymes to tenderize the cut. Meat can be aged no matter how it was raised. Because the process causes the meat to shrink, the price per pound can be significantly higher.

Chicken Stock

Homemade stock brings so much flavor to dishes, I always try to have some on hand.

> 3 to 4 pounds chicken parts (such as wings and legs) and bones
> 1 bouquet garni (bay leaf, sprigs of thyme and parsley, and 6 pepper-corns, tied in a knot of cheesecloth or enclosed in a tea ball) (optional)
> 2 cups vegetable trimmings (such as onion tops, garlic skins, carrot shavings, or parsley stems—avoid any strongly flavored vegetables such as broccoli or cabbage)

Place the chicken and bouquet garni, if using, in a large pot and add cold water to cover by 2 inches. Place over medium heat and bring to a simmer. Reduce the heat to low and continue to cook just under a simmer, skimming any scum that forms on top of the liquid every 20 minutes for the first hour. Do not boil, cover, or stir, or the stock will cloud. After the first hour, remove any whole chicken pieces from the liquid, cool, remove the meat (reserve for another use), and return the bones and skin to the pot. Continue cooking over low heat for a total of at least 3 and up to 8 hours. Two hours before removing from the stove, add the vegetable trimmings to the pot.

When the stock is done, allow it to cool, then strain through a strainer lined with a double thickness of cheesecloth and refrigerate until completely chilled. Remove any fat from the top of the chilled stock. Divide the stock into 1-quart freezer bags and freeze until ready to use.

Makes about two quarts

Eat the Whole Bird

Instead of buying a pound of boneless, skinless chicken breasts, pick up an entire bird. Not only will the cost per pound be lower, you get the added bonus of having not only the two breasts you needed for your recipe but thighs and legs to make another dish and all of the other carcass parts to turn into a terrific stock.

Avoid Boneless, Skinless

Americans are getting more and more separated from the origins of their food, and there is a growing squeamishness about bones and viscera of any sort—of any reminder that the meat was once an animal.[47] It's too bad, because meat that is left on the bone during cooking is more flavorful and retains its structural integrity much better than that which has been deboned. Bone-in meat is also significantly cheaper than its boneless counterpart.

If you need a boneless cut, it isn't hard to do the de-boning yourself. With a little practice, I've been able to save a lot of money by doing so, and always have a bounty of fresh stock on hand from the resulting skin and bones. I learned to do it (and most things in my kitchen) from reading Julia Child's books. She and Jacques Pepin, the renowned chef and cookbook author, demonstrate an easy technique in their video series, *Julia and Jacques Cook at Home*. You can buy or rent this video and follow along. Or check out www.epicurious.com, from the publishers of *Gourmet* magazine, and download a streaming video of the process.

QUESTIONS FOR YOUR
MEAT VENDOR

Which label is best? I wish I had a silver bullet for this problem—one answer that would solve all of the questions. But there isn't one simple answer. The USDA labeling system just doesn't supply enough clear information to make such an evaluation. Some of the best efforts, such as grass-fed meat and heritage breeding, don't always have an easily recognized label. What about the farmers who follow the organic standard—and even go beyond it—but can't afford to file for certification? They shouldn't suffer because they don't have a label. Food production is a complex process and you have to make some judgment calls.

Below are some questions you can ask at the meat counter to make sure you're buying Real Food:

- Are you owned in whole or part by another company?
- What are the animals fed?
- What percentage, if any, of their diet is organic?
- Are the animals subjected to beak clipping/tail docking?
- Are non-therapeutic antibiotics administered?
- Are growth hormones or steroids administered?
- What is the age of the animals at slaughter?
- Are the animals caged?
- Do they have access to outdoors?
- Is rotational grazing practiced?
- How many hours a day do the animals spend outside?
- Who performs or supervises their slaughter?

PROFILE: STAFFORD ENTERPRISES

Honor and dignity may not be the first words that come to mind when you think about a slaughterhouse, but they are the driving forces behind the operation at Stafford Enterprises, a meat processing plant in Stafford Springs, Connecticut. This facility wasn't developed to meet industry standards—although that's something that it does every day, with a USDA inspector on site to guarantee it—it was designed to exceed them. A collaboration of dedicated individuals and associations, including the New England Heritage Breeds Conservancy, Cabbage Hill Farm Foundation, the New England Livestock Alliance (NELA), and consultants such as Temple Grandin, the renowned livestock behaviorist, have collaborated to design this model operation, which seeks to support local family farmers and raise the bar for livestock processing.

The Protocol

At the heart of their efforts is a production protocol that farmers who sell their meat through Stafford must follow. The guidelines, which extend beyond the facility to the field, are something virtually unheard of in the industry, where the concentration is usually strictly results-oriented, with no view toward the path taken to achieve such results. Key points include:

- All animals in the program must be raised in the Northeast, and must be source-verified from birth. They must also be identified with an electronic I.D. tag, enabling consumers to track their meat back from plate to pasture.
- The animals are either totally grass-fed or grass-fed and grain-finished. In both instances, the animals cannot be fed animal by-

products, fish by-products, or bakery by-products, all of which are common in the diets of factory-farmed cattle.

- No artificial hormones or sub-therapeutic antibiotics may be administered to the animals.
- All animals must be handled in accordance with standards set by the Animal Welfare Institute. This extends from their treatment on the farm to the way they are transported and slaughtered,when care must be taken to keep the animals calm and relaxed.
- All animals must be "carcass ultrasounded" at least once. This is a state-of-the-art system whereby the cattle are examined in the field to evaluate tenderness, weight, and stress level.

Benefits

Adherence to the protocol benefits all involved.

THE ANIMALS

Animals that are raised according to the protocol lead low-stress lifestyles. They spend a good part of their life in the fresh air and sunshine. They are fed a natural diet that is easy for them to digest, so sickness and disease is at its lowest. All of the animals raised under NELA standards and brought to Stafford for processing are treated humanely, and all effort is made to reduce the amount of stress they experience from start to finish. When the animals arrive at the plant for processing, every effort is made to keep them calm, such as removing items from the unloading dock that might distract and upset them.

THE EATERS

Happy animals make for happy eaters. The increased health of these animals means that they require less medical treatment, reducing the chance that eaters will be exposed to residue from such therapies. The ultrasound these animals undergo while in the field also ensures good treatment, as it can detect stress in an animal, and guarantees a consistent product—offering a window into the level of marbling of certain cuts.

And unlike the shopping experience at a supermarket, for example, where choice is limited to what is packed in plastic and sitting in the display case, consumers who buy meat from Stafford (from their Web site, www.500farms.com) are offered access to a variety of cuts that meet exacting standards. "The goals at Stafford are to provide a very wholesome, safe, high-quality product to the consumer and give the consumer a choice, and to allow the consumer to know where their meat comes from, to be able to actually know which farm their meat comes from and how it's processed," says Tom Gardner, Founder and President of the New England Heritage Breeds Conservancy and President of NELA.

THE WORKERS

Stafford Enterprises is immaculate, which owes much to the fact that very few animals are processed each day. At larger plants, thousands of animals are processed daily; at Stafford, that number is fewer than twenty. This enables the plant to maintain a rigorous standard of sanitation and safety, which is a plus for workers, animals, and eaters.

THE FARMERS

By following the NELA protocols for raising their cattle, farmers reap many benefits. They are no longer dependent on costly inputs such as chemicals and commercial feed, so their profit margin is higher, and they and their animals can enjoy a better standard of living. And because of the higher premium they are paid, farmers are able to shrink the size of their herds, making life on the farm easier for everyone. As Gardner explains, "The goal is the preservation of small-farm agriculture in the Northeast region. The Stafford processing plant is a critical component in this effort."

You can buy delicious products, pasture-raised on family farms, directly from their Web site.

STAFFORD ENTERPRISES/500 FARMS
30 Furnace Hollow Road
Stafford, Connecticut 06076
Phone: 860-684-0222
www.500farms.com

PROFILE: CABBAGE HILL

Pigs are wonderful mothers. If a hawk is circling above, explains Randy Woodard, greenhouse manager of Cabbage Hill Farm in Mount Kisco, New York, "All the moms will circle the piglets to protect them." He gestures to the creature foraging among bushes, under trees, in and out of a large wooden enclosure. The pig in question is called a Large Black Pig, and is just one of the many rare-breed animals on the farm, also known as heritage breeds. But when Nancy Kohlberg started the farm in 1985, "I always vowed I would never have pigs. I thought they would be smelly and difficult. But I love them now." She discovered that this breed of pig is particularly hardy and requires little care, and the pork produced is "outstanding." Her pigs are not confined—they forage in contentment, and enjoy a life free from stress, particularly compared to the way industrially raised pigs live.

Life at the 170-acre Cabbage Hill Farm is peaceful—Devon cattle wander through rolling pastures and you might spot a Shetland sheep ambling across a meadow. Maran chickens from France peck at the ground, oblivious to the fact that they are among the few of their kind left on earth. Many of the animals populating the farm are endangered, and it is one of Nancy Kohlberg's missions to save them. Early on, she says, "I realized I wanted the farm to have some kind of meaning. I just didn't want it to be an estate. So I really took that idea [of raising rare-breed animals] and ran with it. . . . It grew like topsy."

The farm has grown to include a large greenhouse, which supplies local restaurants with some of the most tender, delicious produce around. "The chef will come over in February, and we'll break out the seed catalogs," Randy Woodard explains. "We custom-grow what they want to put on their plates. . . . It's a really nice relationship. It benefits both of us."

Another instance of a give-and-take relationship exists within the greenhouse itself, where Randy manages an aquaponics system of raising fish. Tilapia, a high-protein, low-fat fish, are raised with no chemicals, hormones, or antibiotics. The water is circulated out of their tanks and used to fertilize the produce grown there. The greens, in turn, act as a filter to the water, which then is cycled back to the fish.

The circle of life is a central theme at Cabbage Hill, and Nancy wanted to make sure that every step along the way was first-rate—from breeding, to raising, all the way to slaughter. But when trying to find a suitable facility for her animals to be processed, Nancy came up empty-handed. "Some slaughterhouses around here are unbelievably bad. I can't believe they're USDA-inspected because they're dirty, they're awful." And so the slaughterhouse in Connecticut she started, Stafford Enterprises, was born. The place illustrates how Nancy believes the final stage of an animal's life should occur—in a clean, compassionate environment. And, unlike most facilities that process animals by thousands, its small scale is geared to the local, independent farmer who is often rejected by facilities that only accept animals in large lots. She hopes it will serve as a model for how a small farmer can avoid "the agribusiness formula," as she describes it, and still thrive.

Survival of the small farm is paramount to Nancy, and she believes its future may lie with rare-breed animal farming. "[These animals] are wonderful for a mom and pop, who might even have jobs during the day. . . . If people would go this route, I think they could save a lot of their properties." Nancy's farm is a working example of how well-suited these animals are to a small farm. "The best thing about these animals is that they require very little care. They like to stay out in all kinds of weather, whether it's the Shetland sheep or the cattle, so there are no barns to muck out. . . . They eat grass in the summer and they eat hay in the winter. They're very hardy. They don't need a lot of supplements. They don't get sick a lot, so there are no antibiotics, and of course we would never consider hormones."

It's vital to preserve these animals, Nancy believes. Industrial ranchers have bred such hardy qualities out of their animals; if heritage breeds were allowed to go extinct, these positive characteristics would be lost forever. She raises heritage breeds as an insurance policy against the fragility of industrial agriculture's monocultured animal breeds. She explains, "All of these animals have a unique gene pool that's very pure, and it's very important to save that. Because if a disease comes, they may be the ones with the pure genetics that might be able to withstand some of these [diseases]."

The animals, the greenhouse, and the slaughterhouse are the first three parts of a four-part equation, the last of which is her restaurant, the Flying Pig in Mount Kisco, New York, named after her beloved pigs. "I realized that small farmers have a terrible time marketing. So I wanted to set an example of how a farmer could hook up with a restaurant." There is a small retail area in the restaurant, as well, where customers can purchase Cabbage Hill meat in addition to food from other local farms.

Nancy Kohlberg is a woman with a mission—or many missions—all of which form a particularly beautiful circle, tracing a line between animal, farmer, chef, and eater. And it's the eater who is perhaps the most tenuous yet vitally important part of that circle—from the diner who enjoys locally produced food at a restaurant like the Flying Pig, or the shopper who chooses grass-fed beef. As Nancy says, the answer to the survival of the small farm and perhaps the survival of the planet "is for people to begin to appreciate good food and healthy food, and know they have to pay more for it." It's up to the eaters, who have the power to make thoughtful decisions with their food dollars, to ensure that, indeed, the circle is never-ending.

CABBAGE HILL FARM
115 Crow Hill Road
Mount Kisco, New York 10549
Phone: 914-241-2658
www.cabbagehillfarm.org

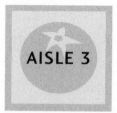

AISLE 3

THE FISHMONGER

'm from Baltimore, where the summer social structure revolves nearly entirely around the catching, steaming, and evening-long affair of meticulously extracting and devouring the meat from dozens of Chesapeake Bay blue crabs. From Memorial Day to Labor Day, you could find my family—three generations of us—lined up at newspaper-covered picnic tables, wooden mallets in hand, waiting for the sharp, vinegary steam to clear so we could crack open the shells, dirty with spices (mustard seed, celery seed, salt, and pepper if my dad was at the helm of the crab pot, Old Bay seasoning if my uncle got his way). Every weekend, the same menu with only two variables. Whose backyard? And, where are we going to get the crabs? Sometimes we'd take the family rowboat out and pull them up one by one using an apparatus with all the complexity of a chicken neck tied to a string. Or, if one of the families we knew in the crabbing business was having a good run, we would help them unload their surplus by buying a bushel or two. Then the air would turn chill, the crabbing season would end, and we would retire our crab mallets until the next season. It was all there—it was local, it was seasonal, it was culturally rich, and it bound our family together.

As I've grown, so has my taste for all things aquatic—not just seafood but the local communities that celebrate it. Fish and chips on the streets of London, chowder in Boston, a good ol' shrimp boil in Baton Rouge, and lobsters in Maine—flavor postcards that I stash in my memory bank, made more vivid by the sights and sounds of the hosting cities. Not just dinners, but tastes of the local culture at its simplest and most delicious. Not that fish doesn't have its merits when eaten with the noblest finery—enrobed in luxurious sauces and nibbled daintily from sterling service; it's just as delicate and succulent when it's dressed to the nines. But it's the intimacy of the tight little food chain—dinner caught, bought, and put in a pot, all in one day, in one community—that makes seafood so alluring to me. It can be the epitome of fresh and local.

INDUSTRIAL AGRICULTURE SNAPSHOT

"Local," however, is becoming an elusive ideal in the seafood industry. My exploration of aquatic edibles and coastal fishing villages turned up some unexpected truths about the state of our waters and its inhabitants. Before I began looking into it, I suppose I thought, more than a bit naively, that anything that came from the wild and raging sea (or even the depths of the murky Chesapeake Bay) was beyond the reach of industrialized agriculture and factory farming. You may be as surprised as I was to discover how closely the underwater food supply mirrors the state of the food chain on land.

A lot has changed since I was at my dad's side, learning how to coax the succulent nuggets of briny white meat from the crab claws he would generously donate to me at the table. The stock of crabs in the Chesapeake

Bay is in big trouble—what was once an abundant, cheap picnic food is now endangered.

Many restaurants have tried to compensate for the low supply by importing cheaper crabs and crabmeat. Unless he reads the fine print, the unsuspecting diner may not know that his crabs have come from other parts of the United States, or that the meat in his crab cake hails from as far away as Thailand. This is dangerous business. Not because I'm a crab snob, which I am, but because it separates eaters from the cyclical nature of the summer crab feast and gives the illusion that all is still right with the crab scene in the Bay—which is anything but true. Crabs are always on the menu (even in December!) so we must have plenty—even more than enough—right?

The globalization of the fish market has managed to veil a lot of the evils of the commercial fishing industry. Now that we can chill, freeze, and transport fish over thousands of miles, fishing need no longer be a local enterprise. According to one estimate, more than 80 percent of the seafood Americans now eat is imported.[1] What used to be a family business that supported local culture and tradition is now, like most food production, the domain of multinational conglomerates who can afford huge fleets of boats that are equipped with sophisticated technology. When they "fish out" one area of the sea, they simply move on to the next. Fish one species to extinction and then create a marketing campaign to push another.

Commercial Fishing Techniques

A sojourn in Halifax, Nova Scotia, opened my eyes to the holocaust humans have inflicted on the marine population. This corner of Canada is renowned for its fish—namely cod—and chips. As I sat at a seaside table, chill wind whipping my napkin away, I set my taste buds on a platter of crispy, fried planks of the area's bounty. When the waitress came to take my order, I asked for the local, fresh catch of the day, expecting the morsels to come from the nets to my plate, nearly flapping from their freshness. She snickered and told me that the only thing "local" on the menu was the beer. I nearly cried when I learned the sad history of this legendary fish—and the even sadder fact that it is a fate shared by many ocean creatures.

Turn back the clock to the 1500s. Cod was so plentiful in the waters off of what is now New England and the Canadian Maritimes that teams of sailors were lured west from Europe by its bounty—cod was one of the main reasons for the French and British settlement of North America.[2] Cod schools were so dense they made navigating the waters a challenge.[3] And now? In certain areas of the Atlantic, cod have been designated commercially extinct.[4] Surprisingly, the waters were fished sustainedly for nearly five hundred years. It has only been since about World War II that, according to the National Audubon's *Seafood Lover's Almanac,* "industrialization of the fishing fleets has outstripped the biological capacity of the fish."[5] The devastation is humbling. Recent studies report that the abundance of large ocean fish—bottom-dwelling groundfish like cod and open-ocean swimmers like tunas, swordfish, marlins, and sharks—has plummeted by 90 percent since industrialized fishing got going after World War II.[6]

How did this happen? The short answer is overfishing. Overfishing, simply put, is catching fish faster than they can reproduce. After World War II, advancements in technology such as sonar equipment allowed fishermen to adopt extremely efficient, mechanized fishing methods. As a result, they were able to catch fish in astounding numbers. Between 1950 and 1994, ocean fishermen increased their catch by 400 percent.[7] The waters just can't support this kind of take. Of the Tokyo fish market, Michael Jenkins, President of Forest Trends, a nonprofit conservation group, says, "It is maybe the biggest fish market in the world, and it's spectacular in its diversity when you look at it, but then you walk away from it, and you think, 'This is unbelievable, this is the bounty of the sea, how much can there be left in the ocean? This is one day, *one* day in Tokyo, is there anything left in the ocean?'" Studies conducted by the Pew Institute for Ocean

Science indicate that the ocean's population is shrinking dramatically. According to them, "Populations of the ocean's top predators—tuna, marlin, and sharks—have fallen to 10 percent of what they were a half century ago."[8]

But overfishing is a complex equation. It's not just the number of fish that are taken from the oceans; it's the way that they are taken. A leading cause of the destruction of wide swaths of marine life and habitats—and the leading cause for the depletion of the Atlantic cod population—is destructive fishing techniques.

Let me explain. Have you ever seen the movie *The Old Man and the Sea*? Just a man, his boat, and a rod and reel. Nice image, but such a scenario is, sadly, mainly the domain of sport-fishermen—those seeking a trophy for their mantle or their fry-pan. Commercial fishing is a whole other story that employs equipment to bring in as many fish as quickly as possible—and often wreaks havoc in the process.

TRAWLING

Trawling is one of the leading offenders in the industry. Large nets, often with weights or tires attached to the bottom of them, are dragged through the water or along the ocean floor to trap fish. This raking action tears up the natural habitats of many animals and gleans the ocean floor of small, fragile creatures that reside in its camouflage until they reach maturity. Cod, for example, keep to the ocean floor for safety until they are large enough to fend for themselves in the waters above. As trawlers rake over the sea floor, they destroy these protective habitats and kill the immature fish. Interrupting the life cycle at this fragile point can lead to rapid depletion of the fishery by killing off, in one pass, an entire generation of young, and with it the fish's capacity to repopulate the waters.

These trawling nets are indiscriminate—they catch anything in their path. This leads to one of the saddest facts of commercial fishing—bycatch. Any marine life that is caught unintentionally is bycatch, and is often tossed unceremoniously back into the water where the process usually kills it. The volume of animal life that is incidentally destroyed in commercial fishing is estimated to be about 25 percent of the boat's take. Animals are discarded as bycatch because there is no market for them, they are illegal to catch—because they are too small, the boat lacks a permit for that species, they are endangered—or they simply weren't the intended catch of the day. Marine animals such as the young of the targeted species (like the cod), whales, dolphins, seals, endangered species like sea turtles, even birds such as the endangered albatross, all die as bycatch. This fishing technique alone takes a tremendous toll on the sea population—and we're not even talking about fish that are eaten.

These other practices, while not as damaging as methods like trawling that scrape the sea floor, also result in large amounts of bycatch:

PURSE SEINING

Two or more boats corral a school of fish by circling it with a net and then drawing the bottom closed to form a huge sort of purse, which is then lifted onto the boat.

GILL NETS

Wide curtains of net are suspended underwater from floats. The net holes are designed to be small enough to let the fish's head through, but not its body. When the snared fish tries to back out of the net, its gills catch on the weave of the net.

LONG LINES

Fishing lines up to fifty miles long are strung with thousands of hooks that are either floated on top of the water or are suspended some distance down.

Toxic Waters

I know when I stand by the sea it makes me feel small, and I imagine that, extrapolated over the population of the planet, that feeling may have a lot to do with the mess that marine life is in. The enormity of the Earth's waters can make the ocean seem invulnerable. It's hard to believe that people, even collectively, could have any power over Poseidon. But in the brief space of time since the dawn of the Industrial Revolution, we have dumped so many toxins into the sea and its many tendrils that there are vast areas of water that are "dead zones"—unable to support any life at all. In the remaining marine population, there is evidence of such high levels of toxicity that the fish are inedible or must play a small role in an eater's diet. I'm not talking about some fish you might hook downstream of the local sewage treatment plant, although that might be unwise as well. I'm talking about the swordfish on the four-star menu, the basket of clam strips from the local seafood shack, and the tuna salad in your lunch bag. All of these items are players in a very sorry fish tale.

Images of polluting companies discharging pipelines of chemicals into nearby waters and headline-making oil spills may be what comes to mind when you think of toxins in the water. These *point sources* of pollution, though devastating, tell only half of the story.

Non-point sources, such as runoff pollution from road surfaces and parking lots, houses, and farms, play an often less attention-grabbing but equal if not greater role in the contamination of our waterways. For example, 50 percent of the thirty-seven million tons of chemical fertilizers used in the United States travels down the Mississippi River.[9] In 1997, a dead zone—an area where toxic agricultural runoff eliminates the water's ability to sustain life—16,000 square kilometers, an area roughly the size of New Jersey, persisted in the Gulf of Mexico.[10] Dead zones are caused by an influx of nitrogen into the water, which triggers dramatic growth of algae or "blooms" that deplete the water of oxygen.

In the lowest concentrations, algae blooms throw a marine ecosystem off balance by denying food or oxygen to strata of the ecosystem. Fish either die from lack of oxygen or move away from the area. In the most severe cases, harmful algae blooms are toxic. You may have heard of Pfiesteria, also called the "cell from hell," which was responsible for massive fish kills and serious human illness (including severe stomach cramps, disorientation, and short-term memory loss among scientists and fishermen who hadn't even ingested any seafood) in North Carolina, and has recently become a problem in Maryland.[11] Although industrial farmers deny any link, the 1995 Pfiesteria bloom in North Carolina occurred after heavy rains washed an estimated twenty-five million gallons of hog waste into the Neuse River.[12] Although the Pocomoke Sound region in Maryland and Virginia is relatively thinly populated, and there is little industry, the area is heavy with poultry farms. As a result, both poultry waste and the phosphate-rich fertilizers derived from it are being studied as possible causes for the spread of Pfiesteria.[13]

Many toxins settle in sediment, where they reach high concentrations that poison the fish that inhabit the sea floor, causing disease, infertility, and death. The major sediment contaminants are synthetic organic chemicals (e.g., PCBs and chlorinated pesticides) and toxic metals (e.g., mercury and cadmium)—the products, by-products, and wastes of industry. Some toxins, such as mercury, do not break down, so they "biomagnify" up the food chain, becoming more concentrated with each fish that is eaten. Larger fish, which consume large amounts of smaller, tainted fish, increase their toxicity levels with each successive meal. As the end point on the food chain, humans are often on the receiving end of the most concentrated doses of toxins when they eat these larger fish or large amounts of the smaller ones.

When I became pregnant with my daughter in 2001, I received a list of "no-nos" from my doctor. I nodded along as he ticked off all of the usual suspects—no alcohol, smoking, easy on the sugar and caffeine. But then he stopped me in my tracks—no shark, swordfish, king mackerel, or tile fish, and limit my intake of tuna and shellfish. He said that the mercury levels in such fish are just too high now to rule out the possibility that they wouldn't contribute to birth defects if I ate them while expecting. I couldn't believe that we had let our waters become so polluted that we couldn't even eat from them safely. I was even more shocked that this was the first I had heard of it. Surely there were kids everywhere knocking back lunch sack after lunch sack of tuna fish sandwiches. What about them?

The FDA and the EPA have since issued advisories to women who are pregnant, may become pregnant, or are nursing, and to small children to limit their intake of certain types of fish (there has been debate between the two agencies regarding the types of fish that should be on the list). As discussed on page 8, the most frightening part of this type of equation for me is that the recommendations are based on averages—the *average* amount of mercury found in a sampling of fish and the *average* level of fish consumption in the population. The reasoning being that, when ingested within the set parameters—only a certain amount over a certain time—the concentration of mercury in the eater's blood will not reach a dangerous level. However, in some fish samples tested, mercury levels were found to be five to nine times above the average.[14] If that happens to be the fish that lands on your plate, you could realistically be consuming more than two months "average" exposure to mercury in one meal! In its 1999/2000 study, the Centers for Disease Control found that 8 percent of women age sixteen to forty-nine tested demonstrated blood levels of mercury exceeding the precautionary standard set by the EPA. The CDC suspects that much of the mercury is accumulated through eating fish.[15]

Farmed Fish

As our waters become more toxic and less bountiful, "aquaculture," also called "fish farming," is a seemingly logical solution to the problems associated with the capture of wild specimens. Fish farming is, in fact, a booming business. The value of farm-raised seafood grew from about $500 million in 1989 to nearly $1 billion in 1998.[16] But ill-conceived factory fish farms make aquaculture a source of significant controversy.

Fish are farmed in one of two kinds of systems: open systems that corral large numbers of fish in pens or ponds in the natural environment, or closed systems that isolate schools in gigantic land-based tanks. Regardless of the setup, fish farming is susceptible to many of the factory farming practices discussed in Aisle 2: The Meat Counter. Like other factory-farmed animals, captive fish are often bred and treated with hormones to grow quickly. And as is the case on land-based feedlots, overcrowding frequently spreads disease, which is treated with vaccines and antibiotics. Disinfectants and herbicides are routinely applied to the inhabited chambers to kill parasites and discourage algae growth.

POLLUTION

The highly concentrated population of factory fish farms, both open and closed, often leads to pollution of the surrounding area. The feed, feed additives, and waste all contribute to the problem.

In open systems, massive quantities of food are poured over floating fish cages, and that which is uneaten falls to the ocean floor, creating a toxic "sludge blanket" under the cage. The fish in the cages create another layer of their own waste, which also winds up on the ocean floor, smothering plant and marine life and poisoning surrounding waters. The quantities of antibiotics, pesticides, and other chemicals fed to and flushed over the fish often leach into the surrounding water and local communities. Closed systems can contain the same toxic cocktail of uneaten food, animal waste, and chemical additives. Powerful filtering systems are often employed to remove these substances from the water. However, improper disposal of removed wastes and periodic flushing of untreated water into surrounding lands and water systems can pollute nearby communities.

AWOL FISH

The fish that are raised in factory farms are often not the same fish you would find in the wild. They are frequently bred for captivity to be slow movers and fast growers. They may be non-native species or the results of experiments to create genetically modified (GM) fish that perform better in captivity. A sad situation in itself, perhaps, but also a threat to the wild population when the farmed fish happen to make their way into open waters. It occurs all too often. On average, 15 percent of farmed fish escape. There are also incidences of mass fish escape. Recently, in

Maine, more than 170,000 farm-raised salmon escaped from a net pen after a storm.[17] The introduction of non-native species and genetically modified fish can obliterate wild populations. Studies show that genetically modified fish are more aggressive, consume more food, and attract more mates than wild fish. These studies also show that although genetically modified fish will attract more mates, their offspring will be less fit and less likely to survive. As a result, some scientists predict that genetically modified fish will cause some species to become extinct within only a few generations.[18]

FEEDING THE FISH FARM

UNNATURAL DIET, INCREASED TOXINS Perhaps you've heard some of the negative press that "dyed salmon" has received. It seems that unlike their wild cousins that feed on shrimp and krill, which give them their famously flame-orange flesh, farmed salmon, because of their diet, have flesh that is notably pale. To compensate, and some would say to bamboozle the eater, farmed salmon is fed enough dye to turn its flesh the customary rosy hue. Much brouhaha has resulted about the nature of the dye and its safety, but I've been left with another thought—what, then (other than the dye, obviously), are they feeding the farmed salmon?

The answer is hauntingly familiar. Just like factory-farmed land animals, factory-farmed fish are fed a concoction that is vastly different from what they would eat in the wild. It includes "forage fish," fish oil, binders and fillers such as soy and corn, and synthetic additives like antibiotics, hormones, and the famed dyes. This diet fails the fish, the eater, and the environment on a number of levels. Fish meal has a much higher concentration of toxins than that of a wild salmon's diet—as a result, farmed salmon have up to ten times the level of PCBs as wild salmon.[19] Farmed salmon is also much lower in the beneficial omega-3 fatty acids that make its wild counterpart such a healthful meal. The great paradox of fish farming, however, is that it actually results in a net protein loss in the sea population. It takes about three pounds of foraged fish to net one pound of farmed fish, so we actually lose more fish than we gain in the process.

VEGETARIAN FEED Herbivorous fish, like catfish, that are raised in closed systems and are fed pellets of soybeans, corn, wheat, and added vitamins and minerals, are often heralded as a fish farming success story—a controlled protein production factory.[20] If you believe, however, as I do, that you are not just what you eat, but you are what you eat *eats,* then the merits of fish farming—even in a closed system—can begin to diminish. As discussed throughout the book, the industrial farming of grains (with its massive amounts of toxins, environmental pollution, and the loss of family farms) is at the root of many of the problems in the American food chain. Feeding these products to fish only extends the associated evils to the sea.

REVIVING REAL FOOD

Like land farmers, generations of families who have passed down a fine stewardship of the waters have been shut out by large companies. Such companies can afford technical equipment and machinery, and can market fish at rock-bottom prices, pricing local fishermen out of the game. But local fishermen are working hard to save their businesses, the seas, and sea animals that are a part of their familial and our collective heritage. They are coming up with creative solutions such as turtle-safe netting, which allows animals to escape the fate of bycatch, and have rejuvenated the population of these endangered species. In Maine, fish farmers are relocating their pens on a regular basis to prevent build-up of toxic sludge on the ocean floor. Sustainable fisheries in California and North Carolina are raising sturgeon, the source of premium caviar, and other egg-bearing fish to halt the rapid decline of the wild Caspian species. As described on page 15, at Cabbage Hill Farm in Mount Kisco, New York, tilapia fish and lettuce greens are raised symbiotically—the fish bring nutrients to the plants and the plants cleanse the water for the fish. A concerted effort between such fishermen, government policy makers, and eaters is the only way for our waters to rebound. Here's what you can do.

Eat Local, Eat Seasonal

I'm not suggesting that you should declare a moratorium on any morsel that did not originate in your neighborhood bog, but it's a good idea to get in touch with the seasonality and state of health of your favorite fish or the fish in your area and to recognize when fish are running plentifully in their native habitats. One of my favorite seafoods, wild salmon, is a summer indulgence. I eat it until it comes out of my ears during the warm months and then hit my frozen stash or lay off as best I can for the rest of the year.

Support Your Local Fisherman or Fishmonger

The best way to stay in touch with the fish supply—local or otherwise—is to develop a good relationship with your local fishmonger. He may not have all of the answers, but starting the dialogue is key. Awareness and sensitivity to these issues is a relatively new thing—don't think that you have to find a new supplier if yours can't list the top most endangered fishes off the top of his or her head. They just might need a catalyst (you!) to get the information ball rolling. If he doesn't have answers to your questions at hand, maybe he will on your next visit, so keep going back.

Know Your Labels

Legislation is underway to change labeling procedures to expand the information available on fish packaging to include, among other things, country of origin. Until then, you really need to trust your source and ask questions. At the end of this chapter are some bullet points you might want to cover in your conversation. And you may not be able to get fish that clears every hurdle. That doesn't mean you have to stop eating seafood. Pick the issue that means the most to you—a fishing method that results in low-level bycatch; wild, not farmed, specimens; or local vs. imported—and eat from there.

FRESH
Fresh fish has never been frozen.

PREVIOUSLY FROZEN
Seafood labeled "previously frozen" is thawed at the store.

F.A.S.
Stands for "frozen at sea." This is the best freezing method, as it retains as much of the integrity of the fish as possible. Some argue that F.A.S. fish is of better quality than fresh fish that has traveled a great distance.

FARMED
According to the USDA's Country of Origin Labelling program (COOL), all fish should be labeled to indicate where and how (whether wild or farmed) it was raised.

CULTURED
Sometimes mollusks like clams, mussels, and oysters are referred to as "cultured" or "cultivated." This is another word for farmed. But because of the way they filter the water for food, mollusks actually clean the water where they are raised, which, it is sometimes argued, is an ecological benefit of such a farm operation. Also because of this filtering process, mollusk eaters must be mindful of the origin of their dinner. Much like a vacuum, mollusks "trap" toxins with their filtering action, so they are only as pure as the water in which they live.

HATCHERY
Hatchery fish are born in captivity, grown to a certain size, and then are released into the wild. While they don't pose the same environmental problems related to open fish farms, they can still stress the wild population by

competing for food and spawning ground and, if they are a non-native introduction, by crossbreeding with native fishes.

WILD

Wild fish is any fish that was born, lived, and is caught in open waters. Not all wild fish are labeled. The exception that I have seen is wild salmon. My market calls a lot of attention to this fish when it is in season, and it is worth every word of its reputation. It is remarkably different from the farmed fish that is available year round. It's bright magenta in color, and when cooked, silky and full of flavor. One taste of this magnificent water dweller wins the farmed vs. wild argument hands down. Additionally, wild salmon, like grass-fed meats (see Aisle 2: The Meat Counter), supplies more omega-3 fatty acids than their farmed counterparts.

Wild Salmon Teriyaki

This recipe not only makes a delicious dinner, the leftovers serve double duty as the base for a second meal of fried rice.

One 2-inch knob fresh ginger
1 to 2 garlic cloves
½ cup soy sauce
½ cup chicken stock (see recipe, page 78) or water
2 tablespoons rice vinegar or white wine vinegar
2 tablespoons blackstrap molasses or honey
1 pinch red pepper flakes (optional)
2 pounds wild salmon fillets
1 teaspoon vegetable oil

Place the ginger, garlic, soy sauce, chicken stock, vinegar, molasses, and red pepper flakes in a blender and puree until smooth. Place the salmon in a nonreactive bowl or casserole just large enough to hold the fish in one layer. Cover with the marinade and refrigerate for 20 minutes, turning the salmon once halfway through.

While fish marinates, preheat the broiler and oil a broiling pan (in place of a broiling pan I use a cake cooling rack that fits neatly into a cookie sheet. The fish doesn't stick to the rack if I oil it well and the cookie sheet catches any drips).

Remove the fish from the marinade and place it skin-side-up on the broiling pan. Broil the fish approximately 4 inches from the broiling element until the skin is crispy and starts to bubble, 7 to 10 minutes. Run a spatula under the fish to loosen it from the rack and flip it over. Broil on the second side until dark brown, another 7 to 10 minutes. Test for doneness by inserting a fork into the center of the fillet. The fish should be opaque and flaky all the way through. If not quite done, turn the broiler off and bake at 425°F until cooked through.

While the fish is broiling, pour the remaining marinade into a small saucepan. Bring to a boil, then simmer for 5 minutes to make a delicious sauce.

Serve the salmon with rice and steamed vegetables and pass the sauce separately on the side.

Serves 4, with leftovers

SURIMI

Surimi is minced white fish that has been washed, strained, and combined with additives, preservatives, and colorants to resemble fresh fish. The technique of making surimi is not new—it has been around for hundreds of years—but has gained new popularity in the sushi market, where it is the primary ingredient in imitation crab meat or "crab stick" and is frequently used in popular California rolls.

Wild Salmon Fried Rice

Fried rice is a perfect second-day meal. You have to use cold rice, or it turns to glue in the pan. So the recycling of last night's salmon feast (or any other rice-based meal, for that matter) isn't just a convenience—it's a delicious necessity!

4 tablespoons peanut oil or other light oil
4 eggs, beaten well
1 yellow onion, diced
2 to 3 scallions, finely chopped
½ cup frozen peas (optional)
Leftover rice, about 2 cups
Salmon, sauce, and steamed vegetables left over from Wild Salmon
    Teriyaki (page 103)

Heat a large nonstick frying pan or wok over medium heat and add 2 tablespoons of the oil. Pour in the eggs and scramble until set. Remove the eggs from the pan to a bowl and wipe the pan with a paper towel. Raise the heat to high, add the remaining 2 tablespoons oil, and heat until hot but not smoking. Add the onion and scallions and sauté until the onion starts to brown, 2 to 3 minutes. Add the peas, if using, and stir until heated through. Break up the leftover rice with your hands (the rice may seem a little dry and stuck together; it will rehydrate and separate when heated) and add to the pan with leftover vegetables and sauce and stir until the rice is coated with sauce and warmed through. Remove from the heat. Add the scrambled egg and salmon and stir to combine. (The heat of the rice will warm the fish without toughening it.) Serve immediately.

Serves 4

TURTLE-SAFE

Turtle-safe nets are specially designed with "escape hatches" that release snared sea turtles back into the wild. Their use is on the rise in shrimp operations whose practices previously threatened the endangered population of these majestic creatures. "Turtle safe" labels, similar to the "dolphin safe" claims on tuna cans, are becoming increasingly evident in the marketplace.

ECOFISH

EcoFish is a New Hampshire–based company that does some of the homework of finding ethical seafood for you by pre-screening fisheries to determine their sustainability. They obtain products that are either wild species, from a healthy fishery caught in an ecologically sound manner, or aquaculture species, from farms that raise their product in a manner friendly to the surrounding environment.

EcoFish supplies restaurants and retailers. Check the freezer case at your local market for their products or log on to www.ecofish.com for a purveyor near you.

Use a Sustainability Guide

A fish species' sustainable status—how abundant or endangered it is—is rarely black-and-white. Some fish are plentiful and well managed on one coast, endangered on another. Fish caught by one method may be a great dinner choice, but when brought to shore by other means may have been part of a destructive scenario that makes them less than appetizing. The following organizations have done a fantastic job of weighing the myriad factors involved when choosing a fish and have rated them accordingly.

AUDUBON LIST

You may think of birds when you think of the National Audubon Society, but the organization offers a terrific wallet card that lists fish on a scale from thriving to threatened. You can download it from their Web site, seafood.audubon.org.

MONTEREY BAY AQUARIUM

The Monterey Bay Aquarium provides region-specific recommendations. You can download their cards at www.montereybayaquarium.com.

SEAFOOD CHOICES ALLIANCE

A comprehensive database, available on their Web site (www.seafood choices.com), compares the recommendations of several organizations and briefly describes the status of many popular fish.

Avoid High Bycatch Fishing Methods

Look instead for individually landed fish caught by rod and reel, pole, or troll-caught. (Not to be confused with trawl-caught—which often dredges the sea floor with weighted nets—trolling is dangling a rod and reel or pole from a moving boat to attract the attention of the fish.) Fish caught in traps is also another good option.

Follow Fish Advisories

Something to be aware of if you are the "catch your own dinner" type. In 2000, 2,242 fish advisories were issued in the United States warning eaters of potential risks of consumption. One might think that this is headline news, but you're not likely to find it on the front page. The place to look is http://map1.epa.gov/ where you can find advisory information for the water you will be fishing and the type of fish you are after.

Eat a Variety of Fish

Whenever a fish becomes popular there is a rush to fill that need, which may strain the population. The Patagonian toothfish thrived in relative obscurity until marketing wizards renamed it Chilean sea bass. Then it flew off menus so fast that the once abundant, but slow to reproduce, species is dwindling to unsafe numbers.

Spread out demand for fashionable fins. Try to be open to suggestions from your fishmonger to try new things that are having a good run or are in season. You don't have to be shy about cooking a new kind of fish—most benefit from a turn under the broiler and a dab of butter and lemon—or ask your fishmonger how he cooks his.

A Special Note About Caviar

Have you tried domestic caviar? Chefs around the country are singing the praises of this tasty alternative to imported eggs. And not a moment too soon. Populations of Caspian Sea sturgeon, which produce beluga caviar, have declined more than 90 percent in the past two decades. Experts believe beluga sturgeon are so depleted that they may no longer be reproducing in the wild.[21] Give these Caspian fish a break by enjoying domestically raised caviar such as white sturgeon, trout, and paddlefish. Log on to www.caviaremptor.org for more info and retail sources. (See the Profile on Sally Eason on page 109 for the story of one such producer.)

Cooking Tips

These techniques reduce the levels of PCBs, dioxins, and other chlorinated chemicals, but not mercury:

- Before cooking, remove the skin, fat, internal organs, the tomally of lobster, and the mustard of crabs, where toxins are more likely to accumulate.[22]
- When cooking, let the fat drain away by grilling or broiling.[23]
- Avoid deep-frying fish, which seals in toxins.[24]

QUESTIONS FOR YOUR FISHMONGER

- Is the fish farmed or wild?
- If farmed, is it vegetarian fish or carnivorous?
- Is the fish from an open or closed system?
- If wild, where was it caught?
- Is it plentiful in that area?
- How was it caught?

PROFILE: SALLY EASON

I'm no stranger to the Carolinas. A large part of my family hails from there, and having spent memorable vacations riding around on tractors and knocking back local pork BBQ and sweet tea, I believed that I had that part of the South pegged. My search for Real Food has taken me on some unexpected turns, but the last thing I thought I'd find in those rolling hills was a forward-thinking caviar producer.

But find her I did. Sally Eason owns and operates Sunburst Trout Company with her husband, Steve, in Canton, North Carolina, in the western part of the state. Sunburst produces a variety of rainbow trout products, notably trout caviar—one of the domestic caviar varieties that Real Food eaters are turning to as an alternative to endangered Caspian roe.

The superb flavor of Sunburst caviar can be attributed in no small part to the meticulous standards under which it is produced. The eggs are carefully harvested only from fish whose skein—the protective sac that contains the eggs—is intact, preserving the delicate texture of the roe. After careful grading and washing, precise amounts of sugar and salt are added to the eggs to cure the caviar and develop its flavor. And, like sustainable land farming, the sustainable aquaculture that Sunburst practices takes great care to protect the local soil and water resources, as well as maintain "clean" fish, meaning that the fish do not receive sub-therapeutic antibiotic or hormone treatments.

"After all," as Sally puts it, "it's all farming, and no matter what you farm, the environment impacts you." The water source for Sunburst's trout ponds is the Pisgah National Forest. The company maintains the integrity of its watershed by using feed that contains no animal by-products and is low in phosphorous, and by removing the solid waste, which is a by-product of aquaculture, from the water that it uses. A customized system turns waste and production scraps into rich compost that is utilized by area farmers and gardeners.

In this budding industry, such hard work is coupled with a great deal of risk. Sunburst's trout, for instance, have to be nurtured for at least two and sometimes three years before they develop the maturity to produce eggs. During this time any number of variables—too much rain, a hot summer—can mean disaster. Sally says, "I know three producers who lost their business because they slept through a rainstorm." In the early years of the company, Sally's husband, Steve, would get up in the middle of the rainiest nights to prevent a malfunction—a broken valve, a covered screen—that might stem the flow of water through the ponds, which is critical to the survival of the fish. Sally says of the business, "It gets in your blood. If it doesn't, you're going to be in trouble. You've got to be in it 24/7."

At Sunburst, raising trout certainly is in the blood. Sally's father, Dick Jennings, founded the company in 1948, calling it the Jennings Trout

Company, on land that had belonged to his grandfather. Sally's sons got started in the business at the tender ages of two and four, when Sally and Steve came upon the two boys covered in the bright orange eggs, spoons in hand. The boys had been tasting the different recipe samples Sally and Steve had brought home for testing and had set aside all but one, which they were happily working their way through. That tot-chosen sample became the standard recipe Sunburst uses for its delectable caviar and Ben, now twenty-four, is the company's chief taster.

Sunburst may be a family affair, but Sally hopes to band together with other domestic caviar producers who share her dedication to quality. The American Caviar Association, which Sally is working to get off the ground, will make domestic caviars more familiar and available to eaters, and encourage shared learning among peers. Sally has already begun such work by touring extensively and leading guided tastings of not only Sunburst's trout caviar but also caviar from other producers who raise different species of fish. This way, eaters can compare the unique characteristics of the different roes. As Sally believes, "Because they have a significantly lower price point than imported varieties, [American caviar] is a more fun product. You can have fun trying the different varieties. Saying here's a lovely trout caviar, but also a great paddlefish [caviar]."

The delectability of domestic caviar might come as a surprise to those accustomed to relying on imports to satisfy their love of the stuff. As may the domestic roe's relatively affordable price—an ounce of Caspian caviar can fetch up to $240, compared to $28 for a two-ounce jar of Sunburst's trout caviar. What has traditionally been considered a luxury product may not be the kind of item that immediately comes to mind when thinking about sustainable farming, but products such as Sally's are proof that cared-for food is first and foremost delicious. Like finding caviar in the middle of BBQ country—such discoveries may surprise and will surely delight.

Domestic caviar such as Sunburst's is available in select restaurants and retail locations. To learn more about Sunburst and sample some of their delicious products, you can contact them directly.

Sunburst Trout Company
128 Raceway Place
Canton, North Carolina 28716
Phone (toll-free): 800-673-3051
Phone (local): 828-648-3010
www.sunbursttrout.com

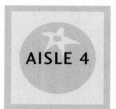

GRAINS, OILS, AND SWEETENERS

I didn't think you could get seasick on land, particularly in the land-locked Midwest. But that was the feeling I had staring out over thousands of planted acres that reached to the horizon. As a passing breeze rippled across the dense fields, my stomach lurched as if I were riding on the high seas. I could almost see whitecaps in the "amber waves of grain." Even though I was looking out onto a vista greatly changed since that patriotic lyric was penned, the inspiration was palpable.

The corresponding images of America's heartland, pure and plentiful, and its residents, families who work the land and work it together, are etched in our collective consciousness. And they are exactly the pictures that I carried in my head when my husband and I set out to cross the United States.

Maybe I had grown up watching a little too much Mayberry, but here's what I expected: farms. Handsome, well-storied, whitewashed houses with wraparound porches like the one my granddaddy grew up in. Surrounded by golden fields dotted with straw-hatted workers tending their plants, maybe stopping to wave at us as we blazed by on our way to town. Local diners serving homemade pies and regular joe. Mom-and-pop grocery stores. 4-H Club fairs.

It appears I showed up a few decades too late. There was mile after mile of crops but a conspicuous absence of human life. From the banks of the Mississippi to the Hoover Dam, I did not see a single farmer in a field. Not one. There were a few lone souls driving tank-sized combines up and down the crop rows. And on more than one occasion, we were buzzed from overhead nearly close enough for a handshake by a low-flying crop duster. But actual farmer-to-dirt contact—I didn't witness it.

INDUSTRIAL AGRICULTURE SNAPSHOT

And now I understand why. "Tending the fields"—which used to entail walking them to determine soil conditions and hoeing them to remove weeds—is now often done remotely and mechanically. Now, I'm not saying that we should return to the backbreaking practices of the pioneers. But the current system of production—which values high volume and profit above all else—has moved so far from the farmer's spirit of land stewardship that it is no longer sustainable for the fields or the grower.

The shift in agricultural values is not so surprising when you see who is at the helm of the industry. The grain-growing scene is commandeered by chemical companies. Dow, Monsanto, and Archer Daniels Midland— the same folks that brought us such lovelies as the pesticide DDT and the herbicide Roundup and are paving the way in many areas of genetic engineering—are calling the shots in the fields and are using their deep corporate pockets to bend farming policy to their will.

The reach of these corporate giants extends further than you might think. The grain crops—dominated by corn, soy, and wheat with cotton, rice, sorghum, and rapeseed (canola) in supporting roles—are the linchpins in our food chain. They are in practically every meal we eat, in all manner of forms and fabrications. They are eaten whole as grains, or in the case of soy, as beans. These crops are ground into the flours that make our breads, cakes, pastas, and tortillas, and are flaked and puffed into our cereal bowls. They are also processed into all kinds of chips and crackers, tofu, miso, and a variety of fillers and binders. And they are pressed and extracted into the majority of our oils and processed into the sweeteners that have become ubiquitous in our foods. Eighty percent of the oil we consume is made from soybeans.[1] The majority of our sugar intake—which adds up to one pound per person every sixty hours![2]—comes from syrups derived from corn.[3] Even a crop such as cotton, something you may not consider an edible commodity, is used in food production for the oil it renders.

Even at that, only a fraction of our grain crops is grown for human consumption. Livestock is on the consuming end of the majority of these crops. In 2003, for example, nearly 60 percent of the 10.2 billion bushels of corn produced in the United States was used to feed livestock.[4]

And grains are becoming increasingly important beyond the kitchen. The grain industry is hard at work to find new applications for these crops. They are used to create textiles, as chemical bases, and as solvents. They can be turned into plastics, alcohol, even wallpaper. The creation of ethanol, a fuel additive, is a growing sector of the corn industry

The promotional campaigns for such products make them sound like an auspicious use of wholesome goods. "Imagine a world that's not diminishing resources, but growing them," says the Archer Daniels Midland (ADM) ad campaign. Corporate agribusinesses rely heavily on the wholesome constructs we all share of the iconic American farming experience and its endless bounty to sell their products and political platforms. Their advertising campaigns flash images of overall-wearing kids in cornfields and weather-worn patriarchs that tap into our collective, if somewhat imagined, memories of farm life that tug on our heartstrings. Without romanticized visions like the ones I had at the beginning of my cross-country journey—full of small-town nostalgia—these corporate goliaths would have nothing on which to base their claim that they are working to save the family farm. Yet the intensive farming of cereal crops couldn't be more damaging.

Monoculture Farming

Of all the planted acres in the United States, more than 80 percent of the fields in 2002 were blanketed with just three crops—corn, soy, and wheat. The majority of cereal crops are raised in monocultures—huge stretches of land planted with the same crop over repeated seasons. Planting in this manner goes against Mother Nature's grain, so to speak.

It's hard to think of water and soil as limited resources, but they are. All farming—digging the soil and irrigating it—requires these natural resources and runs the risk of using more than its share. Freshwater supplies can be contaminated or depleted. Soil can be degraded in a number of ways—through erosion, depletion, and/or compaction. The trick is to strike a balance with the carrying capacity of the land—to take no more than nature can replace. Given the chance, nature has an incredible facility for healing itself, but monoculture farming is so intensive, the environment is constantly losing the battle.

SOIL HEALTH

Untreated soil is not just an inert growing medium, it is alive with millions of worms and other beneficial bugs that aerate it and deposit nutrient-rich, natural fertilizers in it. Crops pull these nutrients from the soil as they grow. After harvest, these nutrients need to be replaced in some way to restore the soil to its nutrient-rich state.

Rather than working with these natural fertilizing agents, farmers who grow monocultures often begin their growing season by "cleaning" their fields—applying heavy doses of chemicals to eliminate any resident insects or vegetation lurking in the plots—and dousing their land with a chemical cocktail to mimic the soil's naturally nutritive state. Regrettably, the pesticides that kill any potentially troublesome insects or weeds also sterilize the soil, eliminating all of the beneficial insects that enrich it. The added chemicals and lack of any vegetation also make the field inhospitable to the winged friends of the farmer, such as birds and bats, that keep harmful infestations in check.

As a result, the fields fall deeper into a catch-22 that requires more chemical applications to patch over the damage caused by the initial treatments. Without beneficial insects, more pesticides need to be applied. The sterilized soil requires the addition of chemical fertilizers for plants to grow in it. It doesn't take long for the crops to become completely dependent on the chemical applications that buttress them.

IRRIGATION

Topically treated fields lack the strong and deep root system that is characteristic of untreated crops that reach into the soil for their strength. Heavy equipment used to apply the chemicals and harvest the crops, as well as the absence of the natural aerating action of beneficial insects, hampers root growth additionally by compacting the soil. Without a rich net of roots to sustain them, these crops are more susceptible to drought and the soil is more vulnerable to erosion.

To compensate for the plants' thirst, fields must be heavily irrigated.[5] This practice uses up valuable sources of fresh water, increases the salinity of the soil, and washes agricultural chemicals into our groundwater and estuaries. Industrial agriculture is draining underground lakes and aquifers faster than they can replenish. Some sources, like the Ogallala aquifer, which underlies 225,000 square miles in the Great Plains region and has been a major source of irrigation for agriculture in the region, are prehistoric sources that cannot be replaced. The draining of such sources is so significant that it is causing land subsidence—the ground is sinking.[6] Surface water sources, such as the Colorado River, have been dammed and redirected to divert water for agriculture, threatening the future of wildlife that depend on them.

Environmentalists claim that a large percentage of the water used in industrialized fields is used wastefully and denigrates not only the water sources, but the land that is irrigated. Excessive irrigation can deposit mineral salts in the soil that can render the land unusable—it's simply too salty to be planted.

Excessive irrigation also contributes to the flow of agricultural chemicals off of the farm.[7] The chemicals leach into our drinking water.[8] According to Environmental Defense, "More than 4 million Americans in 245 communities are exposed to levels of herbicides in drinking water that exceed federal safety standards."[9] The chemicals enter our waterways, where they contaminate wildlife and destroy the natural habitats of many animals, including fish. As discussed in greater detail in Aisle 3: The Fishmonger on page 95, there are entire bodies of water where large volumes of toxic runoff from industrial farms have created "dead zones" that can no longer support aquatic life.

Irrigation and rain also carry the fragile topsoil off of the farm. Some estuaries must be routinely dug out from the large accumulations of farm soil that block their flow. Wind can also blow the fragile layer of soil off of the farm. One of the most horrific examples of this phenomenon was the Dustbowl of the 1930s. After decades of intensive farming and a sustained drought, so much of the topsoil was blown off the fields of the Midwest that home owners on the East Coast were dusting it off of their furniture.

Genetically Modified Organisms (GMOs)

The companies that develop GMOs liken their importance to the creation of fire, and promise nearly as much benefit in the future. They claim that GMO crops will right the wrongs of the industrial agriculture model, that farmers will be able to grow crops in marginal soil that previously could not be cultivated, that such crops will be able to withstand drought and pestilent blight. They assert that GMO crops will be necessary to feed an ever-growing population.

WHAT ARE GMOs?

GMOs, also referred to as genetically engineered (GE), transgenic, or biotech foods, are foods that have been genetically altered, often by the introduction of cross-species DNA at a cellular level. This is not like selective breeding to increase the likelihood of desired traits in successive generations, like planting the seeds from your tastiest tomatoes to get a better fruit—one that is resistant to the pest or climate challenges in your region. Or even crossbreeding, where you might mate a Pekingese and a poodle to have a little "Peek-a-poo." GMO development is often cross-species. It has resulted in sci-fi sounding combinations, such as the introduction of bacteria DNA into plants so they generate their own pesticides, and the splicing of fish genes into tomatoes to make them more cold-resistant.

How do they do it? Once the genes that trigger the desired traits are isolated, they are packaged together with additional genetic material that will facilitate transfer and "markers" that verify the success of the process. This genetic "cassette," as it is called, is then forced into a host by one of a variety of methods. One of the more popular methods for transferring genes from one species to another involves inoculating the host with a bacteria or virus that carries the desired genes. In other instances, the cassette is shot into the host plant with a gun.

The marker gene allows scientists to test for a successful transfer. One of the more common markers is bacteria that has been raised to be antibiotic resistant. To test for a successful transfer, the host plant is fed some of the specific antibiotic. Those cells that survive the antibiotic, because they have been genetically modified to resist it, signify a successful transfer.

The results are unpredictable. In one instance, scientists involved in the genetic engineering of flowers believed their experiment to control the petal color of their plants was successful when the bed burst into glorious white blooms. But they were shocked when a climb in the mercury suddenly turned all of the white posies bright red.

GMOs in use today

There are currently two types of GMO crops that are widely in use—Bt and Roundup Ready. Bt crops generate the naturally occurring pesticide *Bacillus thuringiensis* on a cellular level. That means that these crops produce their own pesticide in every part of the plant—the leaves, stalks, roots, and grains. An insect that ingests the plant material is poisoned by it. Roundup Ready crops are developed by agrichemical giant Monsanto to withstand heavy applications of its popular herbicide, Roundup, without fear of plant damage from overexposure.

Unknown Health Impact The most burning question—Are these crops safe to eat?—goes largely untested. No one seems to know exactly. Some fear that the imprecision of the process could inadvertently raise the toxicity of plants such as potatoes that naturally contain low levels of toxins. Or that toxins such as cyanide, which is formed naturally in the pit of peaches, will leach into the flesh of the fruit when altered genetically. Others contend that crossing the genetic code of various species will cause some eaters to unwittingly ingest known allergens, or that the process will generate new, previously undiscovered allergens. At the very least, some suspect that the nutritional value of GMO foods will be altered.

Unknown Environmental Impact Questions about the impact of GMO crops on the environment also abound. As with most plants, the pollen of GMO plants spreads its genetic code on the wind, allowing such plants to exchange biological information with other plants, insects, and animals. This "genetic drift," as it is called, contaminates non-GMO fields of organic farmers who can no longer sell their crops as GMO-free. Scientists fear that beneficial insects that are an essential link in the food chain may be endangered by encountering GE pollen.

It is widely recognized that heavy applications of pesticides diminish their effectiveness because the pests become resistant to the chemicals. With the concentration of *Bacillus thuringiensis* in Bt-engineered crops such as corn being twenty-five times the concentration of toxin needed to kill almost every pest that might attack a plant, it follows that topical applications of Bt will soon lose their effectiveness.[10] The biotech companies are prepared in such an eventuality, as they always are, to sell farmers the next version of their technology. But the obsolescence of Bt will cripple organic farmers who rely on it—in its non-GMO form—as a valuable weapon against infestation.

The developers of GE seeds claim that their use will reduce the use of pesticides and herbicides in the environment. However, according to the Northwest Science and Environmental Policy Center, the planting of 550 million acres of genetically engineered (GE) corn, soybeans, and cotton in the United States since 1996 has increased pesticide use by about fifty million pounds.[11] Additionally, Bt crops come to our plates with more Bt in the plant than would ever be present from a topical application. How does that reduce residue?

GOVERNMENT "OVERSIGHT" In a splendid example of a governmental hot potato, there is no agency that will take on the responsibility of guaranteeing the safety of Genetically Modified Organisms in our food supply. A policy called "substantial equivalence" essentially claims that because transgenic foods are more similar to their traditional counterparts than they are different, there is no need to verify their safety. For example, if corn is a safe thing to eat and Bt is a safe pesticide to use, then Bt corn, which contains both of these things, must be safe. Without thorough testing, however, there is no sure way of knowing if the whole is the same or different than the sum of its parts.

CERTAIN CERTAINTIES

There may be no clear answers on the health or environmental impact of growing GMO crops, but I don't need a clinical trial to believe that some things are true—that eaters have a right to know what they are eating, and that the expansion of GE agriculture takes too much power away from farmers, the stewards of our land, and puts it into the hands of corporations motivated solely by profits. And I'm not alone in my thinking. The public and professional outcry against GMOs has been deafening and effective. When McDonald's began using Bt potatoes in its french fries, the negative response from their customers was so great that they stopped sourcing them. Without the support of McDonald's, the Bt potato went out of production. And despite the well-funded campaign led by Dow, DuPont, and Monsanto to defeat them, the citizens of Mendocino, California, pushed through legislation to become the first county in the nation to ban GMO crops from being planted within its limits.[12]

HAVE YOU EATEN YOUR GMOs TODAY? Although the act may not have been intentional, chances are the answer is yes. While the GMO debate wages on, millions of eaters, every day, are serving their kids bowls of cereal and knocking back handfuls of chips that, unbeknownst to them, contain GMO ingredients. It is estimated that up to 60 percent of processed foods in the United States have some GE ingredient.[13] More than 35 percent of all corn, 55 percent of all soybeans, and nearly half of all cotton grown in the United States is genetically modified, but to scan the grocery shelves you'd never know it. Paulette Satur of Satur Farms in Cutchogue, New York, observed, "Organic farmers are proud to put the organic label on their products. Why aren't the biotech companies as proud to put a genetically modified label on their products?"

Some people don't like fish. Others eat no red meat. I don't know any cannibals. But if you are eating GMOs, which to date are not labeled, exactly what is on your plate can be very unclear. If plant species are spliced with the DNA of animal proteins, as was the case with some experimental frost-proof tomatoes, eaters will be denied the opportunity to avoid foods to which they are ethically or religiously opposed. One of the scariest turns in the development of GMOs has been bio-pharming—the perpetuation of human proteins, among other pharmaceutical components, in corn crops. Fields, used as giant petri dishes, have been planted with grain spliced with human genes to grow material for use in drug compounds. While never intended for human consumption, it is possible that genetic drift could cause the DNA of such plants to pollinate with neighboring fields where food crops are growing. The resulting grain, when eaten, would result in a form of human cannibalism.

CORPORATE CONTROL Since the beginning of agriculture, farmers have saved, shared, and traded seed. It is a practice that has allowed traits that caused a plant to thrive in the field—resistance to drought or a local pest—or perform well at the table to proliferate. And it saved the farmer a lot of capital for new seed next year.

But by owning the genetic makeup—the seeds—agribusiness holds the genesis of life in its hands. The developers of genetically altered crops patent the plants. This may seem like a formality. After all, who is going to travel from field to field to verify ownership? DNA testing allows GMO developers to verify the presence of the genetic cassette that they implanted and now they are doing just that—traveling farm to farm to enforce their patents and suing farmers into bankruptcy for copyright infringement.

Biotech companies are looking for ways to put an absolute stop to seed saving by producing "terminator technologies" that render the plants sterile and require farmers to purchase new seed with each harvest. Terminator technology has been reviled by world hunger organizations that represent indigenous populations who rely on seed saving to survive.

In a gesture of false altruism, companies such as Monsanto, Syngenta, and DuPont are offering farmers who cannot afford the price of engineered seed low- or no-interest loans to purchase their products. The farmer, reduced to a tenant on his own land, often puts up his farm as collateral to obtain the seed. Should the crop fail, the deed for the land often must be forfeited.[14]

A PLAN FOR WORLD DOMINATION Internationally, the introduction of GMOs into local farming communities reminds many of the Green Revolution of the 1960s, which promised a new agricultural dawn for third-world countries but ended up forcing first-world infrastructure on native populations who could not afford the expensive machinery and costly chemicals on which it relies. Unlike traditional agriculture, which saves seeds from season to season and obtains much of the inputs required for growing, such as animal based fertilizers, from within its own farm system, GMO crops require that new seed be purchased each season along with the necessary chemical inputs they need to grow. Such an arrangement indentures previously independent farmers to the corporations on which they must rely every season for more seed and chemicals. Vandana Shiva, a world-renowned environmental activist, says in her book *Stolen Harvest: The Hijacking of the Global Food Supply*, this shift in power is turning the 70 percent of the world's population that earns its living by producing food from producers into consumers of "corporate-patented agricultural products."[15]

Programs such as Monsanto's "guaranteed market" promise to provide farmers with customers for their grain, but shifting tides in trade policy threaten to topple such arrangements. Some countries allow the import of GMO grains, but others will not even allow the import of products from a country where GMO grains are grown because it cannot be verified that the non-GMO crops were not contaminated by genetic drift or comingled in harvest or transport with GMO material. They also fear that any GMO grain in the shipment might be accidentally planted in their fields and contaminate their own harvests with genetically altered plants.

If GMO crops are adopted on the worldwide level for which agribusiness is striving, the entire globe would be planted with just a few varieties of grain. The abandonment of traditional plant varieties for GMO plants could result in the extinction of a large part of our genetic floral diversity.

Subsidies and Trade

Genetically Modified Organisms are not the only aspect of American farming that is a hotbed of debate. Our subsidy programs, initially enacted to support U.S. farmers against the volatilities of the business, have morphed into a system that often provides more benefit to industrial agribusiness than to family farmers. These programs are often based on principles of increased production that stress the carrying capacity of the land. Because they are awarded to only a narrow selection of crops, subsidies limit the types of grains that farmers can afford to grow. Beyond our borders, American subsidy policy warps prices on the global market, denying many the opportunity to make a living.

SUBSIDIES

If you read the headlines, farming subsidies, government-sponsored programs to support agricultural enterprise, often sound terrific. The PR spin reads like our tax dollars are working hard to support the family farm. And initially, they did provide relief. President Franklin D. Roosevelt's administration designed subsidy programs to stabilize grain prices by buying surplus product from farmers. But in the 1970s, after public outcry during a short-lived spike in grain prices, the government shifted its policy to a subsidy system that paid farmers to quickly increase production.

Lured by the program, some farmers abandoned previously cultivated crops to grow subsidized ones. It's no coincidence that our three largest harvests—corn, soy, and wheat—are also the most heavily subsidized. This has led to a decline in biodiversity, as the variety of crops dwindled, and such an abundance of commodity crops that the prices dropped and have remained low ever since. Market prices are so low, in fact, that they do not equal the costs of production. Farmers operate at a constant loss.[16] Tax dollars are paid to the farmer to make up the difference, but in effect, today's farmer makes less than his father did. For the majority of subsidy recipients, the subsidy program gives them just enough aid to remain viable.

The majority of subsidy money, however, doesn't go to individual farmers—as the policy dictates—but rather to large corporations. According to the Environmental Working Group, which tracks the distribution of such funds, "Today the top 10 percent of American farmers receive 71 percent of the federal subsidy money."[17] And this is just the cash that is doled out directly. Subsidies in the form of reduced-interest loans and discounted infrastructure such as irrigation and drainage also contribute to the bottom line of agricultural support.

These policies, which may sound noble in the headlines (after all, who would want to deny anyone, particularly a farmer, his share of water?), often effect less desirable change when agribusinesses are the recipients. Cheap water, for instance, is leading to the ruination of our water supply discussed on page 117; the government pays for the pipe and the industrial farmers throw open the spigot, at little cost to them but a high price to the environment.[18] The Florida Everglades, for example, one of the richest ecosystems on the planet, was drained in the early 1940s by the Army Corps of Engineers to serve the sugarcane industry. The glades are now about a fifth of their original size and, some fear, irreversibly damaged.[19]

Sugar producers, which include the cane producers of the Southeast and beet sugar farmers in the Midwest, also receive a special kind of economic benefit from government farming policies in the form of input quotas, which are used to artificially raise the cost of sugar in this country. Because we import a minimal amount of sugar, industries that need it to produce their goods must pay three times as much as the going price on the world market. They pass these costs on to eaters, who pay an estimated $2 billion a year extra for their sweets because of this policy.

OVERPRODUCTION Why keep the price of beet and cane sugar so high? Perhaps to force industries to use more abundant forms of sugar, which are the syrups derived from corn, to utilize the growing surplus of that crop in this country. You might think that the fervent production of our grain crops is fueled out of need, that hunger must be driving us toward these ends. But, according to *ABC News*, we grow nearly twice as much corn for the domestic market than we need.[20] As I discuss in Aisle 6: Convenience Foods and Aisle 7: Beverages, the surplus supply of corn in this country is turned into cheap raw ingredients for the processed food and soft drink industries.

Only a sliver of the production of corn, for example, is eaten off of the cob, rolled into a tortilla, or poured into the cereal bowl. The majority, 60 percent in 2001, went to feed livestock.* The rest is processed into "added value" products such as high fructose corn syrup and ethanol, a fuel additive, which brings bigger profits to the producer than using the whole grain does, and, as we'll see in Aisle 6: Convenience Foods, to a large extent, dictates our diet.

TRADE

The rest of our excess production is dumped onto the world market. The practice of "dumping," selling goods on the market at prices below the cost of production to lower market value, is not only illegal, it denies many third-world economies a chance to stabilize, and starves farmers of such countries out of a living. Our trade policies go beyond competition or even capital greed; sometimes they appear to be just plain cruel.

Cotton best exemplifies the nature of such policies. The U.S. government subsidizes cotton so heavily that American taxpayers foot the bill for two-thirds of the costs of growing it.[21] According to the Environmental Working Group, cotton subsidies totaled $10.6 billion between 1995 and 2002, just a shade less than soy.[22] Cotton accounts for only about 5 percent of our planted acres, while soy makes up more than a quarter of them.

Do we do this because without such support we would run out of Levi's? No, there are farmers in Africa who could produce cotton for prices that are a fraction of the actual cost of U.S. production, but their governments can't afford to pay them subsidies, so they have to ask a price that covers their growing. In countries like Burkina Faso in West Africa, historically one of the lowest-cost producers, farmers actually have to pay 10 cents more per kilo than the current price to get product to market.[23]

Some African countries have come to talks sponsored by the World Trade Organization to air their grievances against such policies, but to no avail. The United States and other first-world countries continue to pay

---

*One could argue that feeding grain to animals is using corn for our consumption but, as discussed in Aisle 2: The Meat Counter, feeding ruminants such as cows a grain-based diet is unhealthy for the animal and the eater.

nearly a billion dollars a day to suppress and therefore dominate world markets.[24]

REVIVING REAL FOOD

By holding the reins on our staple crops, agribusinesses control much of our food supply and have a hand in many other facets of our daily lives. Changing the tide of the grain industry, more than in any other grocery aisle, can become a form of political activism. Government policy regarding subsidies is challenged on an international level through the World Trade Organization. At its forums, countries battle for their right to compete on a level playing field. Communities such as Mendocino County, California, have fought and won their right to a GMO-free growing environment, banning such crops within their borders.

You may not see yourself as an activist, but eating can be a political act. Every choice you make in the store supports the efforts of growers who are working outside of the structure of agribusiness. Here's how to cast your vote.

Avoid GMOs

There currently is no labeling requirement for GMO products—companies that use them do not have to declare their content on packaging. Buying products that are labeled GMO-free or that are organic is the only way to be assured that you are not ingesting GMOs.

You may be eating more GMOs—in the form of corn and soy ingredients—than you think, particularly if you eat a lot of processed food. It's loaded with ingredients from these crops. As discussed, corn and soy are some of the most common GMO foods on the shelf. By avoiding them, you can reduce significantly the amount of genetically modified foods in your diet.

But it's not always easy to spot corn and soy products on the shelf.

They may be listed in the ingredients as "corn" or "soy," or they may be called by another name that you might not recognize. Here I've included a list of many corn and soy ingredients—some of which are quite obvious and some that are a bit more obscure. You might be surprised where they turn up—breads, pastas, and cereals, even salad dressings and baby formulas—so be sure to read labels carefully.

CORN PRODUCTS

- Grits
- Polenta
- Corn syrup
- Fructose
- Cornstarch
- Dextrose
- Corn oil

SOY PRODUCTS

- Edamame (large whole soybeans sold in the pod and shelled—seek out organic ones for snacking)
- Hydrolyzed vegetable protein (a flavor enhancer)
- Lecithin (an emulsifier)
- Miso (a salty condiment used in Japanese cuisine)
- Natto (fermented soy condiment)
- Soy isolate (a fibrous soy protein used in food processing)
- Tamari, shoyu, teriyaki (condiments)
- Tempeh (fermented soybean cake)
- Tofu (soybean curd)

Buy Organic Grains, Oils, and Sweeteners

Not only will you be avoiding pesticide residue, but you will be GMO-free.

Because they are single-ingredient items, grains, oils, and sweeteners that are labeled organic follow the same guidelines as whole foods. They are:

- Grown and produced without most conventional pesticides
- Raised without fertilizers that contain synthetic ingredients or sewage sludge
- Not bioengineered
- Not irradiated
- Kept separate from conventional crops during harvesting, processing, transportation, and storage. All equipment that comes in contact with conventional crops must undergo a thorough decontamination before being used with organic crops.

Grain-Specific Ideas

Seek Out Alternative Grains

Food industrialization depends on concentrated demand—millions of eaters lining up to buy the same thing. Take that demand away and you've taken away the incentive from large companies to dominate the production of such a product. As an eater, you can alleviate the pressure on overproduced crops, reduce corporate control of the food chain, and enjoy delicious, meticulously grown "boutique" grains by simply expanding your grain horizons.

Corn, soy, and wheat aren't the only grains out there; they're just the most industrialized. Try out some of the smaller crops—some of which have been around since the time of the pharaohs—as whole grains or processed into breads and cereals, and you will be rewarded with unique flavors and textures. And because these grains are grown on a small scale, they are less likely to succumb to industrialized practices or genetic engineering. Some tasty treats include:

AMARANTH
Originally from Central and South America, amaranth is actually a seed. It is tasty steamed in vegetable or chicken broth then sprinkled with toasted sesame seeds.

COUSCOUS
It isn't actually a grain, but small balls of dried dough similar to pasta. It cooks up quickly, and makes a nice bed for vegetables or a rich sauce.

CRACKED WHEAT
The berries of the wheat broken (cracked) into small bits, are delicious in casseroles or salads and add an interesting texture.

EINKORN
Believed to be one of the oldest grains of all, and as such is the ancestor of all modern wheat. Researchers have found evidence that this grain was present at the very beginning of agriculture.

EMMER WHEAT
First cultivated in Babylonia. It is also called starch wheat or two-grained spelt.

KAMUT
Has a rich, almost buttery flavor. The kernels are large, and it's delicious marinated in a salad. It's also made into flakes and eaten as breakfast cereal.

MILLET
A very mild grain that is easy to digest. It's great prepared as you would rice, but takes on a nuttier flavor if you toast it in a pan (without oil) before boiling.

QUINOA

Quinoa ("keen-wah") is actually a fruit. Thousands of years ago, the Incas considered it sacred. Today quinoa can be found in cereals and baked goods, crackers, cookies, and breads. It is also available in whole-grain, flakes, or flour form. It is wonderful cooked in juice for breakfast. One thing to look out for: The outer part of quinoa is coated with saponin, a bitter tasting substance that protects it in growing but can cause indigestion, so be sure to rinse it well.

Quinoa Salad

The ancient grain quinoa is delicious and unusual, and makes a nice change on the plate from rice or potatoes. It's important to wash quinoa before cooking, as the grains produce a natural detergent, saponin, which is quite bitter.

> 1¼ cups quinoa, washed and drained at least 4 times, until the water runs clear
> ½ teaspoon salt
> 2 tablespoons olive oil
> 2 red peppers, cored, seeded, and julienned
> 1 jalapeño chile, seeded and julienned
> Juice from 1 lime
> 1 teaspoon ground cumin
> ½ teaspoon garlic powder
> ¼ cup chopped fresh cilantro
> 1 small red onion, finely diced

Toast the quinoa in a medium saucepan over medium heat until lightly browned and fragrant. Add 2 cups boiling water and the salt, reduce the heat, and simmer for 15 to 20 minutes. Meanwhile, heat 1 tablespoon of the oil in a large sauté pan over medium heat. Add the red peppers and jalapeños and cook until soft, about 5 to 7 minutes. In a large bowl, whisk together the remaining tablespoon oil, the lime juice, cumin, and garlic powder. Stir in the peppers, cilantro, onion, and quinoa. Serve cold or at room temperature.

Serves 4

SPELT

Often called *farro* in many Italian cookbooks, a distant cousin to modern wheat. Aside from its nutty taste, spelt is particularly nourishing because of its tough husk, which protects it from losing its freshness and nutrients and shields it from pesticides.

TEFF

A tiny grain that has been favored in Ethiopian cooking for thousands of years. It can be white, brown, or red.

TRITICALE

A combination of wheat and rye, formulated in the late 1800s. Many hailed it as a breakthrough because of its higher protein content.

Explore Different Types of Rice

Many of us grew up with just one type of rice—white. This concentration of demand is appealing to agribusinesses that are trying to convert the U.S. rice crops into GMO plantings. Stop them in their tracks by diminishing the demand for this ubiquitous rice. Enjoy a range of varieties instead, such as:

ARBORIO RICE

A type of short-grain rice used to make risotto and paella.

BASMATI RICE

A fragrant hulled long-grain rice from India. It is best when it has been aged for one year, and the label should tell you this.

BROWN RICE

Chewier than white rice, and more nutritious because only its inedible outer husk has been removed, leaving the high-fiber bran coating.

JASMINE RICE

Also hulled and long-grain, and similar in flavor and texture to basmati. It is also fragrant.

TEXMATI RICE

A branded version of basmati rice grown in Texas. It's slightly fluffier and milder than the Indian basmati.

WEHANI RICE

Has a red-colored bran layer. When you cook it, this rice smells like popcorn and tastes slightly sweet.

WILD RICE

Wild rice is actually a type of aquatic grass. It is North America's only native cereal grain. It was and still is considered sacred to area tribes. "Natural" wild rice, such as that found on public waters in Minnesota, is hand harvested. It has to be hand-picked just as the native American Indians did, by knocking the shafts with sticks so that the grains fall into the bottom of the boat. Commercially grown "wild" rice is cultivated in paddies in flooded fields in states such as Minnesota and California and in Canada. It can be harvested with a combine. Ken Goff, executive chef at the Dakota

Bar and Grill in St. Paul, Minnesota, says that while "the cultivated rice is more consistent in taste and color, the lake rice is more delicate."[25]

Where to Find Great Grains and Rices

You may not find all of them in your local grocery, but health food stores and some of the larger organic markets such as Whole Foods carry many of them. Look for family producers, such as the Lundberg family in California, who are growing grains using sustainable methods. Such growers respect the land that they are using, the food they are providing, and the eater who enjoys it.

You also can find other small producers online, such as Native American tribes that are preserving the traditional genetic strains of grains harvested by their ancestors. One such product, Iroquois Corn, is being grown by Pinewoods Community Farming in upstate New York (available through the Bioneers Web site, www.bioneers.org). The corn, rich in history and tradition, is also being recognized throughout the culinary industry as a flavorful addition to the kitchen and has begun popping up on menus nationwide.

A Note About Bread

Describing someone or something as "white bread" is not to pay them a compliment. The food symbolizes the bland, the typical. After all, we're not talking about the creamy white, chewy interior of a French baguette, but the marshmallow-like, presliced, uniform, flavorless loaves that, at their zenith, symbolized America's love for the quick and easy if not the most flavorful choices. Like TV dinners and spaghetti in a can, the factory-fabricated fluff was a staple of the family kitchen. Today, the options for filling one's bread box are much more varied. Whether used as the bookends for some tasty sandwich ingredients, laced with a silky pat of butter and some luscious preserves, or for mopping up those last slurps of stew, real bread is a treat. And now good loaves are readily available no matter where you shop.

ARTISANAL BREAD

Artisanal bread—handmade from start to finish by a trained professional—is as much about the baker as it is about the ingredients. If you've ever tried your hand at bread baking you may have discovered, as I have, that it takes more than the basic elements—flour, water, salt, and yeast or other leavening agent—to turn out something hot and crusty. Innumerable factors—practical ones such as the day's temperature and humidity and less measurable elements such as the feel of the dough—play into the success or failure of every loaf. Only the hands of a master baker can consistently turn out the magical loaves that elevate the bread basket from a device to stave off pre-dinner hunger to something you could make a meal out of. The craft of bread baking, like that of cheesemaking, is gaining strength, making delicious breads more readily available than ever before. If you have a bakery in your town, you might ask if they are handcrafting their own bread. It is also not uncommon to see a range of elegant baguettes, rustic boules, and inviting batards proudly displayed by local bakers at the farmers' market. No matter where you find your artisan bread, stock up. It freezes well when wrapped in foil, then plastic. When you're ready to enjoy it, just remove the plastic and pop the foil-covered loaf in a 350°F oven for 10 to 15 minutes.

PAR-BAKED

Even at the MegaMart, you can often smell the gentle waft of warm loaves emerging from the ovens. Chances are these aromas are from par-baked loaves. Such bread is partially baked and flash-frozen off-site, then shipped to retail locations where they are browned in the store's bakery. There are mixed feelings about such breads among bakers. On the one hand, par-baked breads are made in large quantities, which seems counter to the individual attention upon which artisans pride themselves. On the other hand, the breads are often crafted under the supervision of a master baker, and, since they come out of the ovens throughout the day, the eater gets a fresh loaf that needn't contain any preservatives to prolong shelf life. While I would never want to see the completely handcrafted loaf replaced by such offerings, par-baked breads are a delicious alternative to most packaged breads that you find in the bread aisle, and the variety that they afford eaters—raisin/walnut, ciabatta, sourdough, multigrain, to name a few— makes for delicious opportunities. Many of these breads are sold as whole loaves, but you can have them sliced upon request to a thickness of your choosing—just ask the folks in the bakery department.

PREPACKAGED BREAD

Even among prepackaged loaves, there are gems to be found. While these breads lack the crusty exteriors of fresh baked breads and the varied, crumb (interior) of hand-formed loaves, organic breads, a variety of different flours, such as buckwheat, rye, and spelt, and added grains, seeds, and nuts, have taken sandwich-making to a whole new level. Even whole wheat loaves, once the subversive food of antiestablishment types, have made the leap to the bread aisle at the MegaMart, where they wait sliced, packaged, and ready for their slather of PB and J. While this is good news for eaters, there are some shortcuts being taken, of which you should be aware.

GRAIN SWITCH Some "whole wheat" breads on the shelves actually contain only a small percentage of whole grain flour. Instead, manufacturers use denatured flours—in which the grain's oils and many of its nutrients have been removed—to extend shelf life. To make sure this isn't the case with your loaf, read the ingredients. The first item listed should be "whole wheat flour," not processed ingredients such as "wheat flour," "enriched flour," or "bleached flour," which would indicate a lower percentage of whole wheat in your slice.

ENRICHED BREADS Many prepackaged loaves advertise themselves as "enriched" to project an image of a nutritious product. These breads are made from the denatured flours listed above that have had many of their nutrients removed in the manufacturing process. A fraction of the lost vitamins and minerals are then added back to the flour to "enrich" it.

COLORINGS AND FLAVORINGS Good bread is a beauty to behold but, in prepackaged breads, beauty is often only skin deep. Dark breads, such as whole wheat or pumpernickel, which should get their coloring from the deep tones of their ingredients, sometimes are manufactured with inferior products and then just colored to give them a rich, dark appearance. The appearance of food colorings, often "caramel color," on the label indicate such practices.

Manufacturers of commercially produced breads often sweeten their slices with high fructose corn syrup. As I'll describe in Aisle 7: Beverages, such sugar is a by-product of America's corn glut and has a dubious reputation among health professionals. If you like a slightly sweet loaf, look for breads with a bit of honey or molasses added to the mix.

Oil Ideas

There are a lot of ways to talk about oil. The medical community often talks about saturated and unsaturated fats and those that are high or low in cholesterol to address issues relevant to health. Chefs speak of high and low smoke or flash points—the amount of heat an oil can take before it smokes and eventually bursts into flames on the stovetop.

When I am in the kitchen, I am looking for an oil that has gone through the very least amount of processing. Nutritionists continue to debate the merits or lack thereof in our edible oil selections, but no matter the standard by which an oil is judged, intense processing is bound to degrade it. I look for oils that are the closest to their original sources. I often rely on my senses, rather than information on the label alone, to make my oil selections. I enjoy the characteristic flavors that less refined oils bring to my dishes.

Avoid Chemically Extracted, Highly Refined Oils

There are two major distinctions in oil processing—oil that is derived by chemical extraction and that which comes from mechanical pressing. Chemical extraction uses solvents to break down the oil and remove it from its vegetable source. It is used when the oil component isn't readily accessible, in such plants as soy and corn, or when the producer is looking for a highly cost-effective means of production where the end flavor is of little consequence, as in low-grade olive oil, for example.

Both methods heat the oil to some degree during production. But the thermometer of the chemical extraction process can reach 400°F, which breaks down oils obtained this way.

After being separated from their source, chemically processed oils are then bleached, degummed, and deodorized, often to remove signs of rancidity that result from their high heat production methods. The end result, while highly shelf-stable and heat-tolerant, bears no resemblance to the original form.

Popular examples of chemically extracted, highly refined oil include corn, soy, and canola (rapeseed), which are often genetically modified, and cottonseed and peanut oils.

Seek Out Mechanically Pressed, Unrefined Oils

Mechanical extraction involves pressing or grinding items such as nuts and olives to coax the oil away from the plant matter. "Cold pressed" or "expeller pressed" are terms used to describe oils that are obtained mechanically without the addition of heat, other than that generated by the grinding action itself, to expedite the oil removal. Such methods of extraction are the gentlest, leaving the flavor and nutritional value of the product intact.

Mechanically pressed oil is often left unrefined. It is more fragile than highly refined oil but is prized as the superior product by eaters because it retains more of the flavor and character of the fruit from which it originated. Some unrefined oils are not filtered. Such oil, which hasn't been strained of fine particulate matter, may appear cloudy, but that does not reflect a degradation in quality.

Some of the most popular mechanically pressed oils include safflower, sunflower, sesame (light or dark, depending on whether the seeds were toasted before pressing), and flax seed. These oils must be treated gently. Keep them refrigerated if possible, or at the least in a cool, dark place.

The most popular of the pressed oils, however, is olive. The olive oil industry is largely unregulated, so much of the terminology that is used within it is under little if any scrutiny. Scrupulous producers are working hard to rectify the situation—to bring the same kind of certification standards to oil production that are enforced in the wine industry, for example. (See the Profile on page 146 for the story of one such producer, McEvoy Ranch.)

When shopping for olive oil, look for virgin or extra-virgin, which are obtained strictly through mechanical processes. The classifications describe the oil's acidity—extra-virgin is the most rare, with 1 percent or less acidity, virgin olive oil has 2 percent, and ordinary virgin has no more then 3.3 percent. The very best of these oils are labeled "estate grown," which means that all of the oil in the bottle comes from fruit grown on a single farm. Avoid anything labeled "refined" or "pure." These oils have been treated with chemical solvents after pressing to reduce acidity. They may have been blended with other oils. "Light" olive oil has no official definition. Its light description refers to flavor and color, not caloric content.

Avoid Partially Hydrogenated Oil

Partially hydrogenated oil is processed to carry an extra hydrogen atom, turning it from a liquid to a solid. It is the main ingredient in margarines and spreads and shortenings such as Crisco. As I will discuss on page 183, such oil is widely used in processed foods—as a butter substitute in everything from cookies, crackers, and cakes, and as a frying medium in fast food. Its use is so pervasive in such foods that if you aren't doing the cooking yourself, chances are that you are ingesting it. The process increases volume and shelf-stability but has been linked to health risks so numerous—heart disease, cancer, even neurological dysfunction in children—that it has been banned in some European Union countries. In 2006 it will be under mandatory labeling in the United States.

Return to Animal and Tropical Fats

Animal and tropical fats have been maligned in the past as detrimental to one's health. However, these fats are coming back into favor in the medical community as valid alternatives to partially hydrogenated oils.

Animal fats are obtained by rendering oil from the carcass, or by extracting it from the animal's milk. Fats such as lard (rendered pig fat), tallow (rendered beef or lamb fat), chicken fat (also called schmaltz), and goose and duck fats were, at one time, widely used in cooking and essential to frying and baking. And ethnic cooks and many chefs continue to use such fats in their kitchens to achieve deliciously flaky pie crusts and crispy tortillas, among other dishes.

Another alternative, often used in sautéing, is ghee. Similar to clarified butter, ghee has had the milk fat removed from it to enable it to reach a high temperature before burning. It is often used in Indian cooking and is an excellent alternative to processed oils. You may find it on the grocery's shelves bottled and unrefrigerated.

Tropical fats are being rediscovered for their antioxidant properties. These fats include palm oil (from the oil palm fruit), one of the most important edible oils in the world, as it can be hand harvested and processed on a small scale, as well as palm kernel oil, coconut oil, and cocoa butter, the latter of which is essential in the chocolate industry.

And don't forget about butter. Delicious and satisfying, I'll take a pat of this over a pound of the fake stuff any day.

When Choosing Any Oil

Sometimes label information can be lacking or confusing when selecting an oil. Don't be afraid to fall back on your instincts and your senses and look for the following:

SMELL
The oil should smell pleasant, at least, and at best should give some whiff of the source—the olives from which it was pressed or the sesame seeds that were ground to produce it, for example.

COLOR
A tint of the original source is a good sign in my book. Amber, brown, and emerald green tell me that the product I'm pouring wasn't bleached.

TURBIDITY
An unrefined oil is often a little cloudy. Don't be put off by that. If the oil is within its freshness date, if it has one, or smells fresh, a bit of cloudiness, particularly at the bottom of the bottle where sediment settles, shouldn't be a concern.

OIL SOURCE
Think of the origin of the oil. Does it come from something that you consider oily? I try to stick to oils from foods like sesame seeds that, if pressed between my thumb and finger, would release a little oil naturally.

Sweeteners

When eaters refer to "refined" sugar, they generally mean the white stuff you find in crystals, cubes, and powders. While that sugar is highly refined, other sugars that do not share its snowy white appearance come from the same origins—derived from sugarcane and sugar beets—and are part of the same refinement process or are by-products of it. Turbinado sugar is often called "raw" or "unrefined" sugar; it is actually sugar that has gone through two of the three cycles of washing and crystallizing that are used to produce white sugar. Molasses is a by-product of the refinement of sugarcane (beet sugar molasses is unpalatable; it is fed to animals). It comes in three varieties, "light," from the first stage of refining, "dark," from the second, and "blackstrap," a bitter molasses from the last stage of sugar refinement. Brown sugar is refined white sugar that has been sprayed with molasses to give it a darker color and richer flavor.

Corn syrup is another highly refined product that is used almost exclusively in packaged foods and soft drinks (see page 216) as a less expensive alternative to beet and cane sugars. You also can find bottles of both the light and dark varieties in the market.

Explore Alternative Sweeteners

These sweeteners are made from other plant sources and bring with them unique flavor characteristics. They are not derived from surplus crops, so they do not receive federal subsidies. Also, because they are manufactured in such small quantities relative to cane, beet, and corn sugars, they are less likely to stress the environment through monoculture farming and GMO development.

AMASAKE
Made from fermented sweet brown rice, from Japan. The thick, creamy liquid can be used as a sweetener in cooking or baking.

BROWN RICE SYRUP
Made from sprouted brown rice. It is thick and mild flavored.

DATE SUGAR
A powder made from dried ground dates.

JAGGERY SUGAR
Made in rural India by boiling down the sap of sugarcane or sugar palm trees at a high temperature to give it a rich flavor and dark color.

RAPADURA
Rapadura is the brand name for a sweetener produced by squeezing, drying, and grinding organic Brazilian sugarcane. This process does not separate the sugar from its molasses content, which occurs in the production of refined white sugar, thereby retaining much of the sugarcane's nutrients. It has a mild flavor and is especially good for baking.

STEVIA
From a South American plant whose leaf is said to be three hundred times sweeter than cane sugar, or sucrose. It is not absorbed through the digestive tract and is therefore non-caloric.

Avoid Artificial Sweeteners

I can't think of a single good thing to say about those little blue, pink, and yellow packets stuffed into the sugar bowl of every diner and four-star restaurant. They're just full of chemistry.

ASPARTAME
Marketed as NutraSweet and Equal, it is made up of three chemicals: aspartic acid, phenylalanine, and methanol.

SACCHARINE
Marketed as Sweet'n Low, saccharine is three hundred times sweeter than sugar. Its possible link to cancer has kept saccharine at the center of controversy for many years.

SUCRALOSE

Marketed as Splenda, sucralose is produced by chlorinating sugar (sucrose). It is six hundred to one thousand times sweeter than table sugar. New on the market, it has undergone relatively little testing for safety.

Adopt a New Sugar Strategy

You can steer away from subsidized sugars, such as corn products and cane and beet sugars, by using honey or maple syrup to sweeten your tooth.

The age-old processes by which these products are made reflect a unique relationship between humans and nature. The golden "food of the gods," as the ancient Egyptians viewed honey, is delicately teased from the hives of bees. And, with a bucket and a spigot, the makings of rich maple syrup pours from the trees that dot the Northeast landscape. Many farmers have found these gifts from nature a delicious reward from the land that can also yield an additional income stream.

In small-scale honey production, bees do most of the work, flying about and extracting nectar from flower blossoms then turning it into honey. The source of the nectar determines the particular characteristics of the honey. You can find varieties such as clover, lavender, and orange blossom, which bring a distinctive taste of their floral background to the table and are worth seeking out. On a commercial scale, however, honey is usually made from bees that have been fed sugar water, and accordingly, the honey tastes simply sweet, like refined white sugar, so try to find a small producer for a bigger flavor punch.

Maple syrup is collected by the same means that Native Americans used hundreds of years ago. In late winter and early spring, the sweetwater sap of dormant sugar maple or black maple trees is extracted through tap holes. This sap is then boiled down into a syrup. It takes about forty gallons of sap to make one gallon of maple syrup. There are four grades of maple syrup (Grade A, Grade A medium, Grade A dark, and Grade B), which range from those with a mild flavor and light color to those syrups of the darkest color and strongest flavor, similar to that of molasses. While Grade A is often the most expensive, I opt for Grade B, which has a richer, more "maple-y" flavor.

ISSUES TO CONSIDER WHEN SHOPPING FOR GRAINS, OILS, AND SWEETENERS

- Is the product organic?
- How much has it been refined?
- Is it from a small or large producer?

PROFILE: McEVOY RANCH

Imagine a farm so distinctive you don't need directions to find it. Driving toward Petaluma, California, I spotted one such place—so well-tended and beautifully arranged that it looked like a scene from a movie depicting the Tuscan countryside. I was thrilled to discover that what I was looking at was the very farm I was scheduled to visit. McEvoy Ranch looks as though someone painted it onto the landscape, olive trees lining the gently rolling hills, stretching out like rows of satin trim on the hem of a ballgown. Tidy gardens surround neat buildings, creating an atmosphere of serenity that complements, rather than clashes with, the surrounding landscape. McEvoy strives for this effect, as their Web site explains, continually searching to find "how can the Ranch operation fit more harmoniously within the wild landscape it occupies."[26]

But McEvoy Ranch is far more than just a pretty picture: The 550-acre property produces some of the finest olive oil in the country. It won the

California Olive Oil Council Certification Seal award in 2004, and has gained a devoted following of eaters, chefs, and critics who prize it for its deep, complex flavor and the fact that it is produced organically.

From the start, it was important to founder Nan McEvoy that her ranch be organic, not for certification reasons or even to adhere to the time-honored traditions of olive growing. But because her grandchildren would be visiting often, and she wanted the family to be able to enjoy the splendid outdoor space without fear of pesticides being sprayed that day, or other contact they might have with chemicals. With an eye to integrity—to the land and those that inhabit it—Nan planted her first trees, imported from Tuscany, in 1992. She hired a consultant from Italy to help her implement some of the traditional methods of producing superior oil.

At McEvoy, the olives are hand picked or carefully harvested with a pneumatic combing device, a far cry from many producers who allow overripe fruit to fall to the ground, where it is sucked up into a large, vacuum-like machine before an often long and damaging journey to the mill. McEvoy olives don't travel far at all, since there is a mill, or "frantoio," as it is called in Italian, on the property. Having a mill on-site is essential to the production of quality oil, says Shari DeJoseph, orchard manager at the ranch. "When Nan was planning this whole venture, and working with our Italian consultant, Maurizio, he definitely stressed the point that if she wanted to make high-quality olive oil you had to have your own press, so that you have complete control." With the frantoio on-site, the fruit makes it from tree to press within hours—before any of its vital, flavorful components break down.

The ranch is home to six different varieties of Tuscan olive trees, and, as in their native Italy, the fruit is picked early and green. "We want our [fruit] to have the very peppery, pungent, olive flavor to it, so we know that we need to get it picked before it has a certain percentage of color to it. . . . We would get more oil if we waited later, but because we want that very peppery flavor to the oil, we're sacrificing quantity for the flavor, for the quality that we want," says DeJoseph. McEvoy olive oil does produce somewhat of a "bite" in the back of the throat, a flavor that differs from what many eaters are used to, but one that they would do well to appreciate. Researchers have discovered that such a sensation indicates that the oil is full of healthful polyphenols and antioxidants, which ward off cancer and balance good and bad cholesterol.[27]

A key part of the McEvoy mission is to make consumers and other farmers aware of what good olive oil should taste like. "This style of olive oil requires educating the public, because it's a style that Americans are not used to. They're used to a much more mild, sweet, bland olive oil," says DeJoseph, describing an expectation of taste that has made it that much easier for producers to get away with combining a small amount of extra-virgin olive oil with refined oil to produce an oil that is neither as healthful nor as flavorful as great olive oil should be. "American palates are not developed," says Michael Coon, McEvoy's sales and marketing manager. "People have either had really bad oil, or not cared for it properly. Nan wants the industry to be as serious as the wine industry."[28] The ranch has tastings at their retail store in San Francisco and works closely with their extension agent to share information with other growers.

In addition to producing high-quality olive oil, McEvoy Ranch is a wonderful example of sustainable agriculture at its best. The ranch embodies a closed circle of production, wherein little is wasted and quality reigns supreme. The ranch uses water from its own lakes to drip-irrigate the olive trees, and has an extensive composting operation. A significant portion of the mowing is done with the help of a neighbor's sheep, letting the animals graze to their heart's content in the spring, when the ground might be too wet for a tractor to navigate. And, as DeJoseph explains, one of the "side benefits of having the sheep here to keep the grass down is that they're fertilizing as well." Even the gophers that inhabit the place— usually cursed and expelled from a farm—are appreciated for the fact that they aerate the soil.

The self-sufficient philosophy of McEvoy brings economic benefits as well. Because it's organic, the ranch requires little in the way of purchased inputs such as pesticides and synthetic fertilizers. And with their own mill, McEvoy doesn't have to pay a third party to have the fruit pressed or expend excess fossil fuel to get their olives somewhere else to be processed, as many growers do. When new trees are needed—either for the ranch itself or for sale to other producers—they are propagated in the ranch's nursery, and the circle continues.

From the production of olive oil several other branches of enterprise have grown, further contributing to the self-sustaining system of the ranch. "Nan wants to see that diversity," says DeJoseph. "That keeps the place exciting for her." McEvoy makes and sells soap, hand salve, and other olive oil–related products, and there are plans to harvest honey from the ranch's own hives. A one-acre garden planted with treats that range from figs to fennel supplies chef Gerald Gass, who often prepares staff meals from the bounty that grows just outside his kitchen door.

Not that they're in it purely for the food. Because it's such a great place to work, most of the employees have been around since the beginning and have no intention of leaving. "That stability always helps in the long run, instead of having constant changes," says DeJoseph. As on most farms, important information is always being passed down, often orally, and when such information is lost, the farm suffers. The knowledge that DeJoseph herself brings to McEvoy Ranch is vital to its success: "I've seen these trees grown over ten years, and agriculture is very site-specific. . . . For a perennial crop like this, you need some years of history of the plant to know how they've done, what you've done to improve their health, what's helped them out, what hasn't helped them out."

To many people, the olive branch is a symbol of peace and abundance, and McEvoy Ranch exemplifies these qualities. Simply wandering through the rows and rows of trees, surrounded by the gorgeous California countryside, or perhaps watching a rabbit on a romp through the hills, is bucolic bliss. A salad over which McEvoy oil has been drizzled bursts with exquisite flavor. The demand for quality over quantity, the determination to live in harmony with the surrounding natural beauty, and the careful and sustainable use of the land all stand as signposts that modern agriculture would be wise to follow.

McEvoy Ranch
P.O. Box 341
Petaluma, California 94953
Phone: 866-617-6779
www.mcevoyranch.com

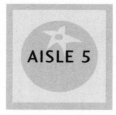

DAIRY

There is perhaps no other foodstuff that lends itself as readily to sheer alchemy as milk. Whether it is from cow, sheep, or goat (even yak!), milk can be separated, aged, cultured, and flavored into all manner of edibles. Luscious cream and butter, tangy yogurts, crème fraîche, and diverse cheeses all get their start at the udder. Even in its liquid state, milk dons a variety of cloaks—from skim and reduced fat, to full fat and even chocolate—to suit the palate of the eater.

And from where I sit—on the receiving end of the fork—lovingly prepared dairy items from an attentively run farm are one of the supreme delights of the table. And, along with eggs still warm from the nest, they offer the eater a direct connection to farm, farmer, and animal that is unique to the dairy aisle. Their high level of perishability behooves us to seek out the freshest product—and our efforts are abundantly rewarded. The smell of fresh butter sizzling in a hot pan or my preferred dessert, the after-dinner cheese course, are culinary delights that can only be realized when products are nurtured from farm to fork.

When I was growing up, I didn't know cheese—not real cheese. I don't think many people in this country did in the early 1970s. Cheese was something that came wrapped in plastic and lasted for months in the refrigerator. It was available in three varieties: yellow American, white mozzarella, and bright pink dotted with nuts—an exotic treat reserved for special occasions. And it had very little to do with the rich and diverse delectables Europeans have been churning out for centuries.

I wish I could say I had that one revelatory moment—my dairy "Aha!" But it was more gradual than that—a taste of farmhouse cheddar on a school trip to Vermont, the tang of cultured butter on my first trip to France, real cream in my coffee. All baby steps that have led me to seek out the boldest, "smells-up-the-whole-fridge," authentic cheeses, and to carry individually swaddled fresh eggs home from the farm. Long gone are my "individually wrapped slices" days. Now it's all about the individual producers, herds, and processes that never cease to carry me to the next level of my flavor odyssey. Fortunately for eaters, there's a legion of such producers gathering strength in our midst. (See the Profile on page 173 for the story of one such producer, Cowgirl Creamery.)

INDUSTRIAL AGRICULTURE SNAPSHOT

Processed cheese items were a boon to companies that manufactured them, such as Kraft. They lasted forever on display and in the fridge, and were cheap to produce—using ingredients, such as milk protein concentrate (MPC), an inexpensive imported powder derived from skim milk.

Manufactured cheese-like objects, like many of the dairy items on the supermarket shelves—such as milk and cream, butter, yogurt, even eggs— are the products of a factory farming system that parallels the absurd practices—including overcrowding and hormone and antibiotic usage— of meat production in this country. And this kind of production is propped up by tax dollars and government supports similar to those inherent in the grain industry.

Like meat and grain production, dairying requires a high level of infrastructure to deliver product from farm to table. Unlike produce, which can be sold as it is harvested, dairy commonly undergoes treatments such as pasteurization and homogenization before it reaches your market. The cost of these processes is most easily borne for conventional milk producers by large operations that can cover expenses through large production volume. Small producers that can't afford such a setup are often forced to sell their raw milk to a large operation that can process it for market or find a creative way to make a profit in this highly pressured industry.

The price for liquid milk is kept so low that it is sometimes more cost-effective for a farmer to stop farming than to continue his business. Some dairymen and women have found that consolidation of the dairy industry and overregulation—which can cost the farmer tens of thousands of dollars in redundant inspection processes and mandatory marketing fees that fund such programs as the "Got Milk?" campaign—have simply made it impossible to make a living on the farm. For others it has forced them to adopt factory farming practices that provide the razor-thin profit margin that allows them to hold on to their farms.

Factory Dairying

Milk- and egg-producing female animals are raised under intense conditions to maximize production and efficiency. Like other factory-farmed animals, dairy cows are fed a grain-based diet that is ill-suited to their digestive systems, often sickening them, and can contain all manner of food industry waste—orange peelings, bakery refuse, scraps that are often laden with pesticide residue and other chemicals. In an effort to economize, egg-laying chickens are sometimes fed rendered proteins from butchered cows, and it is common to feed cows "chicken litter," the detritus of feathers, excrement, and uneaten feed that falls to the bottom of chicken cages. (Although feeding cows rendered cow protein has been banned, feeding them this litter presents a loophole for this type of cannibalism, which has been linked to the transmission of mad cow disease.)

Although administering artificial hormones to poultry has been banned, their egg production is increased by other means. They are subjected to light therapy that extends their laying season beyond their natural cycle, which wanes in the winter months, giving their bodies a rest to recharge. It has become standard practice to starve chickens for one to two weeks toward the end of their production cycles to cause a "forced molt," which triggers the laying of an additional round of eggs—a practice that compromises the bird's immune system and causes increased incidence of salmonella contamination.[1]

Milk production is increased by administering a genetically engineered version of BST, a naturally occurring bovine hormone, to the herd. These genetically modified hormones, also known as Posilac, rBGH, and rBST, were developed exclusively by the biotech company Monsanto. They have been on the market since 1994 and are currently used in about a third of the nation's nine million dairy cows.[2]

There is a great deal of controversy surrounding the use of artificial growth hormones in the dairy industry. Skeptics suspect that cows treated with such inputs produce milk that is chemically and nutritionally different from the milk of untreated cows, that such milk poses health risks to humans, and that the growth hormones are passed through the milk. They cite studies that note an increase of IGF-1, which has been linked to breast and gastrointestinal cancer, in the milk of cows treated with synthetic hormones as a possible health risk to dairy eaters.[3] Critics also point to the increased rate of mastitis, an udder infection that results from the increased milking schedule; it leaches pus into the milk, and requires a course of antibiotics to treat the ailment.

Yet Monsanto relentlessly contends that milk from cows treated with the artificial hormones they produce is no different from that of untreated animals. They have even gone so far as to sue organic dairies and others for simply labeling their products as being free of artificial hormones.[4]

The argument over the effects of artificial hormone treatment in dairy cattle is a moot point. We simply don't need it. We have such an abundance of milk in this country that in the 1980s the government paid farmers to *stop* milking. They offered dairy farmers a lump sum buyout to stop dairying for at least five years in an effort to reduce the glut. Today, there remains such a surplus of milk that farmers who wish to stay in business often rely on federal subsidies to make ends meet.

But the intensity of the industrial practices continues to escalate. Cows and chickens subjected to such a system are quickly spent, living only a fraction of the lifespan they would enjoy under more suitable conditions. Chickens who are relentlessly required to lay eggs soon are sapped of all their calcium stores and their bones become so fragile that they break under their own weight. Cows are crippled by the constant treading on cement floors and the weight of their bloated udders. These depleted animals are then sold into the meat market. The chickens are too bruised to be sold at the retail level—they are often used in processed food where their appearance won't be noticed. The cows are turned into the nation's hamburger supply.

REVIVING REAL FOOD

Our collective taste buds are drawing us back to a more sensible and delicious dairy system. It's not so much a new way of doing things as it is going back to raising animals with respect and showing a dedication to wholesome, traditional practices. It wasn't long ago—not more than fifty years—that all dairy products were organic. Pesticides were not yet the rage. There were no artificial hormones to pump up production. When you poured a glass of milk you knew just what was in it—milk, sometimes a little chocolate if you were lucky, but that was it, no hidden surprises. While the debate over the use of these chemicals wages on, many eaters are choosing to enjoy the tried and true, "all milk" version of the beverage. Dairy is the most rapidly growing segment of the organic foods revolution.[5] Given that children drink the most moo juice, it makes sense to err on the safe side. Organic dairies shun the use of artificial hormones and feed their animals a diet of organic fodder that is pesticide-free.

Other farms, such as Straus Family Creamery in Marin County, California, go beyond organic by pasturing their herd. These cows are allowed to roam on lush paddocks of grass and legumes—a practice as old as milking, with many benefits. This natural diet is agreeable to their systems, so there is less sickness in the herd and, therefore, no need for antibiotic treatments. Unlike the concentrated reservoirs of waste that collect on an industrial dairy farm, the cows' movement across the fields distributes their waste over a wide area where it breaks down naturally, enriching the soil. The farmers' chores are lessened. They no longer need to purchase, store, and haul large quantities of expensive grain. And, with the cows in the field, their clean-up duties are greatly reduced.

And it's terrific for the eater. Milk, like meat, from grass-fed animals is rich in conjugated linoleic acid (CLA), which shows promise of reducing the risk of cancer, obesity, diabetes, and a number of immune disorders, and may even aid in weight loss.[6] The rich milk from these animals is top-rate, reflecting all of the character of the animals' upbringing, their surroundings, and the changing seasons. This high-quality milk is delicious in the glass and lends itself to silky creams, unctuous yogurts, and butter so rich that producers claim it nearly churns itself.

A contingent of dedicated farmers—of cows, goats, and sheep—are opting to perform the alchemy of the creamery entirely in-house. Rather than selling all of their milk for processing, these farmers take on the role of artisanal producer themselves, turning all or part of their milk into products such as butter, cream, yogurt, and cheese, even ice cream. Single-herd operations, such as Ronnybrook in Ancramdale, New York, use only the milk from cows on their farm to create yogurt, crème fraîche, ice cream, butter, and, seasonally, egg nog. Other creameries, such as Straus, team up with neighboring farms that adhere to the same principles of land stewardship to produce a range of dairy products. Some creameries are having great success with other animals. Coach Farm, in Pine Plains, New

York, for instance, transforms its goat's milk into acclaimed yogurts and cheeses, and the Old Chatham Sheepherding Company, in Old Chatham, New York, does the same with the milk from its sheep herd. In-house processing allows these farmers to increase their revenue by adding value to the milk they produce and gives them total control over the quality of the final product.

Symbiotic loyalty is developing between the new dairy farmers and their growing population of loyal customers. Farmers are striving to raise the bar of flavor, and eaters are building new roads to greet them. Here's how to get your good stuff.

Milk

Buy Local Milk

Milk is a living thing, full of natural enzymes that give it flavor and the ability to become cheese. The trend in milk processing, however, is to remove this natural magic so that milk has the transportability, shelf life, and, I would argue, flavor, of bottled water. California leads the nation, as it does in the majority of agriculture output, in milk production. There simply is no need to transport milk thousands of miles across the country. Vermont cows are just as good at producing the stuff as their West Coast counterparts—even better, Vermonters might argue. Seek out local milk and you will be saving us all the needless expense of transporting such goods.

You might also find that the milk tastes better, fresher. That's because milk that is shipped long distances is often ultra-pasteurized—heated at a higher temperature and/or for a longer time—than milk that is simply pasteurized to extend its shelf life.

Pasteurized milk is heated to 145°F (62.8°C) for half an hour or 161°F (72.8°C) for fifteen seconds. This heating kills most, but not all, bacteria in the milk. The shelf life of such milk is twelve to sixteen days under normal refrigeration (below 45°F). *Ultra-pasteurized* milk is heated to a minimum of 280°F (141°C) for two seconds. The resulting product can be stored under refrigeration for thirty to ninety days.[7] This process kills virtually all of the bacteria in milk but results in a "cooked" taste when compared to less processed milks. At the extreme end of the milk-processing spectrum is boxed milk. It is ultra-pasteurized, packaged in a sterile environment, and sealed in an aseptic (sterile and sealed) package. It needn't be refrigerated until opened, which makes it convenient to stock in your pantry shelves, but such convenience comes at the price of flavor. I wouldn't use this stuff for anything more than lightening coffee.

Cooperative markets and independent groceries are often good sources for local dairy. It's not uncommon for them to broker with area dairies for fresh milk and other items. To identify local milk, look at the packaging. You should see the name of the farm or at least the region of the point of origin on the carton.

Buy Regional Milk

Even at area MegaMarts, you can pick up brands such as Organic Valley, which have united local family farmers and sell their milk in localized regions to avoid extensive shipping. Organic Valley offers farmers who opt out of conventional dairy practices a market for their product and take away the advertising and distributing burden that can cripple a small operation. And they pay producers a premium for milk that adheres to their standards, giving the farmer a better shot at earning a living.

Consider Raw Milk

When I was a kid, my grandparents used to squirt freshly drawn milk straight from the udder into the waiting mouths of the barn kittens and any kid who had the skill to catch it. My grandparents didn't even give it a second thought. We all enjoyed the lovely fresh milk, its cream rising to the top of the jug, every day without incident. Today, my grandparents would be thought outlaws.

Raw milk—bottled as it comes from the cow, unpasteurized and non-homogenized—is illegal in many states. Yet there are advocates, such as Sally Fallon of the Weston A. Price Foundation, who argue that with all of the enzymes intact, raw milk is a more flavorful and healthful product. She claims that pasteurization halts enzymatic activity and actually makes milk more likely to be a vector for food-borne illness than carefully produced, well-refrigerated milk that has these natural pathogenic defenders intact. And that the lack of homogenization—left to settle, the fat of raw milk rises to the top of the bottle, creating a thick floating layer of cream and leaving behind naturally low-fat milk to drink—results in a more heart-healthy product.

I think that, like all Real Food, you have to consider the source. I, for one, would not be keen to knock back a glass of untreated milk from an intensive farming operation. But I love cheese made with care from fresh, raw milk and I'll take a glass from a happy cow and clean pail any day—I'll even still try that udder trick. (See www.realmilk.com or www.weston aprice.org for more information about this debate.)

The growing number of dairy drinkers interested in raw milk is using direct purchasing to obtain their coveted unpasteurized product. Gleta Martin and Tim Wightman, owners of Clearview Acres, a Wisconsin dairy farm, began a cow-sharing program to sell raw milk directly to consumers through a loophole of ownership that allowed them to do so legally. By operating in this way, eaters get to enjoy a product that they believe is better nutritionally, and farmers get to develop a direct relationship with their clientele and retain a much larger percentage of the profit from sales of their goods. The program allowed the debt-strapped Clearview Acres operation to increase its income by one-third. Gleta Martin said, "It was the most wonderful thing that ever happened" in her twenty-seven-year career on the farm.[8]

Look for Organic Milk

Choosing organic milk helps reduce pesticide usage, antibiotics, and hormones, but keep in mind that organic is not the last word in quality eating. Like conventional milk, organic milk may have been ultra-pasteurized and shipped across the country to your market. Additionally, many organic cows are raised in the same type of factory-farming systems that produce nonorganic dairy products. Wayne Hansen, who with his wife, Marilyn, owns Wayne's Organic Garden, in Oneco, Connecticut, told me the story of an organic farm that he visited. It was a brand new dairy farm, and the owner guided Wayne through the extensive (and expensive) new facilities. The farmer was telling Wayne all about the "organicness" of his operation and was showing off all the stainless steel and polish of the very well-organized layout. Then he opened the back door and off in the distance were row upon row of broken-down shacks—the shantytown that was the province of those who worked on the farm. It is this kind of disparity that breaks the hearts of many involved in organic food.

That being said, an organic seal guarantees eaters that:

- The milk comes from cows that are fed an entirely organic diet, free from animal by-products.
- Any pasture in which the animals are allowed to graze must be untreated by chemical applications.
- The cows can never be treated with antibiotics or hormones.
- The cows may never be administered or fed genetically modified material of any kind.

Try Some Other Animal Milks

The milk from animals such as goats and sheep provides an alternative to those who are sensitive to cow's milk. Some eaters who cannot digest cow's milk find that they can enjoy goat's milk and goat's milk products such as cheese and yogurt. Such milks have distinctive tastes that some drinkers love, and others don't care for. Decide for yourself. You can find such products at health food stores and national chains such as Whole Foods.

What About Plant-Based Milks?

These "milks," which include soy, rice, and almond, are creamy liquids made by extracting compounds from these grains and nuts. Because they are lactose- and casein-free and are derived from nonanimal sources, they are often used as substitutes for animal's milk by those who are intolerant or avoid animal products for ethical reasons. They are often available in regular and low-fat varieties and a variety of flavors, and some brands are fortified with calcium, vitamin D, and/or vitamin B_{12}.

Soy milk is at the center of a great deal of debate, particularly if it is given to children as a beverage or in infant formula. Proponents argue that drinking the milk of another animal is unnatural and that soy milk offers a wholesome alternative source of nutrition. However, studies have shown that the isoflavins in soy milk mimic the body's natural hormone secretions so closely they can cause health problems when ingested in significant amounts. Additionally, the majority of soy products are genetically engineered—a process with unknown health and environmental impacts. If you are going to buy soy milk, make sure it's organic—it's the only way to ensure you aren't drinking GMOs.

Ice Cream

You might not expect it, but the frozen treat aisle is a great place to find Real Food. Ice cream made with organic and Fair Trade ingredients and without artificial ingredients or flavorings is available nationally. Often local or regional brands such as Brigham's in New England and Straus Family Creamery on the West Coast are also represented. You can often find such items wherever you shop.

I am from the Julia Child school of thought regarding butter. A little is good, a lot is better. Butter, of course, is only as good as the milk from which it is derived. So when I am looking for good butter—and there are dramatic differences in flavor and texture—I look for the same things that I enjoy in good milk. I want the stuff to be from unmedicated animals that, preferably, have some access to pasture. And I want the finished product to be as unadulterated as possible, with no flavorings or additives to mask its rich, full flavor.

Such products are not popular in the MegaMart where fake, oil-based "butters" line the dairy case and high-priced "luxury" items, such as whipped butter, charge eaters for the introduction of air into their toast topper. I stock up my freezer with a few pounds of good butter at a time from "better grocery stores" such as my local health food stores, private groceries, and national chains such as Whole Foods. Here are the hallmarks of good butter:

Buy Organic

As in all other categories of food, I buy organic to avoid exposure to toxins. The same holds true with butter. And, as in milk, it's also my guarantee that I won't be introducing artificial hormones into my diet.

Try Cultured, Also Called "European Style," Butter

I use these butters when I really want to feature butter as a major player in a dish—in a butter sauce or served at room temperature with fresh radishes and salt for dipping. Typically the product of small-batch production, cultured butter has been inoculated with enzymes so that the lactic acid develops, like yogurt. This process gives the butter a slight tang, so it has more character than industrially produced butters. It often has a higher fat content (about 86 percent as opposed to the USDA minimum of 80 percent) than mass-produced butter, resulting in a creamier texture and increased malleability that is favored by chefs. Because such butters are generally produced by artisans who meticulously monitor the health of their herd, I am less concerned about this category of food being certified organic.

No Flavorings, Please

Salt can be introduced as a preservative or to mask substandard quality. Typically, salted butter contains roughly 2 percent salt to give it extra flavor. Chefs and serious cooks usually avoid it as an inferior product to unsalted butter—its salinity can throw off the flavoring of a recipe. Lightly salted butters (in the range of .3 percent salt), which give a subtle counterpoint of salinity to the butter without masking its flavor or disturbing recipe measurements, are sometimes available.

Avoid "Fake Butter"

Butter-flavored spreads, sprays, and margarines are the most egregious example of smoke and mirrors in the grocery aisles. Although they take up the better part of the real estate in the butter section of the refrigerator case, most of them are so loaded with chemicals and preservatives that they needn't be chilled. Buy them and you are paying for chemically flavored hydrogenated oils. The hydrogenation process turns these liquid fats—most frequently corn and soy oils—into solids, and is the main culprit in the preponderance of the widely maligned trans fats in our diets. (See page 184 for further discussion of the link between trans fats and disease.) Because these fats are based on corn and soy products, they are likely to contain Genetically Modified Organisms (GMOs).

In addition to the "butter" flavoring that gives the tasteless oils their palate-fooling profile, variations made "with olive oil," or "with yogurt" also line the shelves. These products try to cash in on the favorable properties of items like olive oil and yogurt by broadcasting such ingredients on their labels. A closer examination of the ingredient list reveals that such ingredients make up a very small portion of the recipe for these products; they are largely used merely as flavorings in a hydrogenated oil base.

"Calorie-free" sprays take advantage of a little labeling loophole that allows them to lay on their "skinny" claims. In fact, the product contains as many calories as any other bottle of flavored oil and water. But because they have such low calorie count per serving (typically one spritz) the caloric content is not required to be listed.

On occasion, butter does make its way into these fake products in limited amounts. "Soft baking butter," for example, is not actually butter alone but a mixture of butter and oil. The oil content allows this product to maintain a spreadable texture even when cold. "Light" butter typically has had air or water introduced into it to lower the caloric value of each portion.

Yogurt

If I can think of one product that holds all of the connotations of "eating well" or "healthful eating," it would be yogurt. The creamy concoction has become synonymous with wholesome food. Moms spoon it into baby mouths. Health-conscious eaters use it as an ingredient substitute in everything from muffins to milkshakes. And its reputation is largely well deserved. The live active cultures it contains—the probiotic bacteria that give yogurt its tang—have been associated with everything from good digestive health to decreasing the risks of some cancers.

Unfortunately, manufacturers, in the interest of gaining market share, have introduced a wide variety of additives to yogurt, taking it very far from its humble, unflavored state. Scan the yogurt section of the dairy aisle and you're likely to see so many variations on the yogurt theme—no-fat, low-fat, cream on the top, with fruit on the bottom, blended with fruit, with granola, with sprinkles—that finding just plain yogurt sometimes can be a tall order. Here's how to separate the goodness from the gimmicks.

Buy Organic, But . . .

When buying yogurt, by all means seek out organic varieties. But read the labels. Even organic yogurts can contain loads of sugar and thickeners. Instead, buy plain, unflavored, unthickened yogurt and stir in some fresh fruit or a tablespoon or so of preserves for flavor and sweetness if you like.

Avoid Bangles and Beads

Steer clear of highly colored yogurt products or those that come with candy on the top. These tricks have been adopted by the industry to entice young eaters, and it just sends the wrong message to your kids. Good food should be valued on its quality, not its ability to turn your tongue purple.

Cheese

There is only one strategy for eating good cheese, and that's to eat real cheese. Not cheese that has the "Real" seal on it—that only guarantees that a product contains at least 51 percent of a dairy component (butter, cheese, or milk) made from cow's milk produced in the United States. By real I mean cheese that is produced on a relatively small scale under the supervision of an artisan who takes care and pride in their work, often utilizing age-old techniques.

When I buy such cheeses, I don't concern myself so much with finding organic products. Good cheesemakers are so particular about the milk they use that I trust them to police the herds with more zeal than any label could guarantee.

Don't be afraid of cheese that comes from unpasteurized milk. In the United States, the terms "unpasteurized" or "raw milk" cheese often put eaters off. Perhaps they think that the product is dirty, or maybe it's our history of eating antiseptic appearing cheeses such as Velveeta that has added to the cultural aversion. The government's regulations, that all raw milk cheese be aged for at least sixty days and that expectant mothers should avoid all such products entirely, add to the view that these items are somewhat dangerous. But the sixty days aging gives raw milk cheese plenty of time to develop the beneficial enzymes that keep it stable. And European cheeses have been made with unpasteurized milk since the beginning of the craft. Not just funky, small-batch stinkers but widely popular varieties such as Parmigiano Reggiano and some Swiss cheeses such as Emmenthaler are made from raw milk and are delicious because of it.

Find a Cheese Shop

The best way to procure real cheese is through a good cheesemonger. Such shops portion cheese to order, they don't sell too many prepackaged wedges, and will allow you to taste before you buy. They are also fountains of information. I can spend the day at my local cheese shop, Darien Cheese & Fine Foods (www.dariencheese.com); they have a story for every item they carry, and I am an eager pupil. (See their Profile on page 176.)

But you don't have to sign up for the complete education plan if that's not your bag. Just tell the proprietor what you want—something creamy to put on a sandwich, a nutty thing that melts easily, or a couple of treats that will finish off a nice meal—and they will be happy to fill your requests and give you as much or as little detail as you're up for.

Look for an Active Counter

If you don't have a cheese shop in your area, you still can find some good cheese at the market. To hedge your bets against getting less than nice cheese, look for a cheese section that has a lot of turnover; cheese that is wrapped for too long will suffocate and go off. If you can find a manned counter, all the better. Ask that person what has just been put on display.

Scout Out a Producer

Cheesemakers often set up a stall at the local farmers' market. They are a great resource for artisanal, local products.

Shop Online

Many independent creameries do mail order. You won't be able to taste before you buy, but you can get a terrific amount of information by ordering directly from the producer. Many offer discounts for large orders to offset the shipping costs, so consider hooking up with a friend or two to realize some economy. Better yet, throw a cheese-tasting party and turn your buddies on to quality dairy delicacies.

Look for a Contact Number

If you find a cheese that you like in your market, look for an Internet address or phone number on the package and don't hesitate to follow up with questions. Artisanal producers are eager to share their stories.

Try Sheep's Milk and Goat's Milk Cheese

If you haven't already, give these non-cow cheeses a try. They are produced on a smaller scale than many cow's milk cheeses so you'll be taking the pressure off of cow herds to keep up the volume. And they have a wonderful, earthy flavor.

Buy Whole Cheese Cuts, Not Shreds or Slices

Buy whole cheese cuts and shred, slice, or grate them yourself to maintain freshness and flavor and avoid anti-caking additives.

Avoid Processed Cheeses

Processed cheese foods are products that have a cheese base but have colors, flavors, and other additives to make them more meltable or spreadable. They must contain 51 percent cheese by weight. Processed cheese products, such as Kraft Singles, do not contain cheese. They are made from powders and oils that imitate a dairy flavor.

Eggs

There is a lot of confusion around the labeling of eggs. Many of the descriptors you see emblazoned on your carton are unregulated. Those that are defined by the USDA, such as free-range, are defined so vaguely that producers with less than honorable intentions still can use them to describe factory-farmed products. Even the USDA Organic label, which strictly details the types of feed and vet care that a bird can receive, requires only access to the outdoors, with no specific regulation of the time, if any, actually spent there. Egg farmers who are raising their laying hens humanely—on nutritious feed and with the adequate space and light that lets a chicken act like a chicken—may have something good to crow about, but are left with few clear labeling choices to separate them from their industrialized competitors.

The best way to get the backstory on your omelette is to do a little research yourself. Producers who are proud of what they are doing are more than happy to show it off. Many put an Internet address on the side of the carton so you can see pictures of their farms and read about their farming practices. Or you can ask your market manager about the eggs they carry. They might have some brochures to share with you or the numbers where you can reach the farms. Talking to the farmer is really the best way to get the lowdown.

Pastured Eggs—The Gold Standard

Pastured chickens spend some portion of their life in the barnyard or field scratching for grubs and insects and supplementing their diet with some greenery. Their diet is completed with some grain, so ask your producer if his feed is organic. The consumption of field greens, which are high in beta carotene, gives the yolks of pastured eggs a bright saffron color and an incredibly fresh taste, and makes them better for you. A SARE- (the USDA's Sustainable Agriculture and Research Education Program) funded study found that such eggs had 10 percent less total fat, 40 percent more vitamin A, 400 percent more omega-3s, and 34 percent less cholesterol.[9]

Because of the chickens' dependence on fresh grass, the pastured eggs they produce are seasonal—you won't find them in the winter. They are largely the dominion of small producers who sell them directly to chefs and eaters, so check your local farmers' market for a supplier near you. Shake the hand of an egg farmer. Treat yourself to real farm fresh eggs.

It's a great weekend tradition to ride to the farm and pick them up. Or grab them at your local farmstand, farmers' market, or co-op.

Warm Lentil Salad with Poached Eggs

This recipe takes eggs off the a.m. shift and puts them on the dinner menu. It calls for French lentils, or lentils du puy. They are available in health food stores and better markets. Don't substitute any other lentil variety—they don't hold their shape as well.

1 pound lentils du puy, rinsed and picked over for small stones
5 strips bacon (preferably organic or grass-fed)
1 medium yellow onion, finely diced
2 garlic cloves, minced
1 teaspoon dry mustard
1 cup dry white wine
2 splashes Worcestershire sauce
2 teaspoons white wine vinegar
1 tablespoon Dijon mustard
Salt and freshly ground black pepper
1/2 cup high-quality olive oil
1/4 cup chopped fresh parsley
1 bunch bitter greens, such as watercress, chopped (optional)
8 eggs, poached, fried, or boiled

Place the lentils in a medium pot, add water to cover by 3 inches, and bring to a boil over high heat. Reduce the heat and simmer, uncovered, until the lentils are tender and some have begun to burst open, 20 to 30 minutes. (Cooking time may vary; check the lentils every 5 minutes after the first 15 minutes of cooking.) Drain.

While lentils are cooking, place the bacon in a large heavy-bottomed skillet over medium heat and fry until crisp. Remove the bacon to a double thickness of paper towels to drain and reserve. Add the onion to the bacon fat in the pan and sauté until translucent, 5 to 7 minutes. Add the garlic and dry mustard and sauté 1 minute, until fragrant. Add the wine and reduce until thick and syrupy, about 5 minutes. Remove the pan from the heat. Add the Worcestershire sauce, vinegar, Dijon mustard, and salt and pepper to taste, and whisk to combine. Slowly drizzle in the oil, whisking constantly to make a vinaigrette. Add the lentils and parsley to the pan and toss to coat with dressing. Crumble the reserved bacon and toss it over the lentils.

Serve the lentils on a bed of bitter greens, if using, topped with poached, fried, or boiled eggs.

Serves 4, with leftovers

Know Your Labels

OMEGA-3 EGGS

These come from chickens that have been fed flax seed to mimic the omega-3 fatty acid content of pastured eggs. Omega-3, which has been related to reduced risk of cancer, can also be found in walnuts and coldwater fish such as salmon, or by eating flax seeds or their oil directly.

ORGANIC

The organic standard, as it applies to eggs:

- Guarantees that the birds are fed an all-organic diet that contains no animal by-products or GMO ingredients
- Does not imply that the animals are raised out-of-doors

"VEG-A-FED"

The birds are fed an all-vegetarian diet that contains no animal by-products. The grain is not necessarily organic.

CAGE-FREE, UNCAGED, FREE-WALKING

Laying hens are raised without cages. However, there may be ten thousand of them in a hangar.

FREE-RANGE, FREE-RANGING

According to the USDA, free-range animals must have access to the outdoors, but producers do not have to guarantee that they use it. Leaving the hangar door open, for example, qualifies chickens as free-range, even if they never cross the threshold.

NATURAL

Not treated with chemicals after harvesting.

FARM FRESH

The only way to find farm fresh eggs is to have some connection to the farm—either a direct relationship with a farmer or a trusted third party, like a co-op manager, operating on your behalf.

QUESTIONS FOR YOUR DAIRY PURVEYOR

- Is this product local?
- Does it come from a single farm? Cooperative? Conventional operation?
- Was the animal pastured?
- Is this product organic?
- Is the item pasteurized? Homogenized?

PROFILE: COWGIRL CREAMERY

Something delicious is happening in a renovated hay barn on a quiet street in Point Reyes, California. Sue Conley and Peggy Smith, self-described "cowgirls," are producing some of the best cheese in the world. In addition to their own Cowgirl Creamery, the barn houses a gourmet deli, a local weaver, and an organic produce stand. This rustic arena, Tomales Bay Foods, is the marketplace and distribution vehicle Sue and Peggy created to promote and sell the agricultural products of Marin County. "The idea of this is so people can actually taste the products they pass that are growing in the fields," Sue explains. "We're not only promoting our own cheeses. And I think that makes us unique. And that's why restaurant chefs want to work with us. They want to have that good, fresh cheese that we make and they want to know what else is going on."

In the dappled sunlight that filters through the century-old beams of the barn, several just-made creamy mounds are lined up in front of a display case, where beautifully wrapped disks of cheese are waiting to be bought by a lucky eater and perhaps spread on a crusty baguette from Brickmaiden Breads, the hearth next door. Or simply nibbled on their own, perhaps with a glass of wine, preferably local wine from the selection available at the neighboring stall. It is this synergy of local efforts that is the manifesto of Tomales Bay Foods and the driving force of its founder.

"I'm an entrepreneur and love building a business," Sue explains, "so that's how this idea was formed. Initially it was just a marketing group called Tomales Bay Foods that identified this place, Tomales Bay, with fine dairies, because we really do have some of the best milk in California. We've got the cool, coastal breezes, and the long growing season for the grasses, a very nice environment for the cattle, and a market fifty miles from here that's the best market in the world for this kind of stuff." Sue loved the cheese that she was helping to promote so much that she decided to become a cheesemaker herself, and Cowgirl Creamery was born. She hooked up with a local organic dairy, Straus Family Creamery, and her cheese is made from their milk exclusively.

Artisanal cheeses like Sue's are handmade in small batches, and the people who put in the long hours to produce them are craftspeople, using traditional methods with care and dedication to quality. Cowgirl's cheeses are rich and complex, and have garnered national awards; one selection, Red Hawk, was described by one judge at the Best of Show competition run by the American Cheese Society as "a breakthrough in American cheesemaking," while another dubbed it "simply sublime."[10]

And cheesemakers like Sue, with her commitment to organic ingredients and traditional artisan practices, also represent a growing movement away from industrial agriculture. The combination of Cowgirl Creamery and Straus Family Creamery is an example of sustainable agriculture at its best, using the land in a responsible, thoughtful way to produce delicious, handcrafted food. It is this connection of cheesemaking to the larger picture of agriculture as a whole that led Sue beyond working as lead cheesemaker to the business of how agriculture and a sustainable environment can coexist in peace. She is on the board of the Marin Agricultural Land Trust (M.A.L.T.), which works to help farmers keep their land by purchasing conservation easements from landowners. Sue also works with several other groups to foster cooperation between the two sides, like the county agriculture commission and the extension office. "One thing about Marin County is that we have a collaboration between environmentalists and agriculturists that's not seen in most areas," Sue explains. "Everyone's at the table. . . . Environmentalists are usually single-issue organizations— they're trying to save the fish, or improve the water quality, or whatever, and that will specifically affect one or two farms. So where these [farmers] have been practicing [agriculture] in a certain manner for a hundred years on the same land, then there's all of a sudden a problem with the way they're doing it because of a new environmental law or a new organization. . . . What we try to do here is not have laws that these guys can't comply with, but to work with them to make it better."

And her efforts are paying off. She's worked with the county to establish an education program for both farmers and consumers that transitions farmers into organic agriculture, and has developed a label, "Marin Organic," to inform eaters that products are both local and organic. "Even though we're a bunch of Berkeley hippies," she says, "these ranchers love us. They really appreciate us, and we really appreciate them, too. They understand that we are here to help. The hardest part for farmers, and it always has been, is figuring out how to work together. . . . They're out there on their own trying to slug it out, and unless you're of a certain size, you just can't do it."

Even with her eye on the bigger picture, Sue's focus on producing delicious, highest-quality cheese never wavers. "I love cheese and the cheese world, too. It's really full of eccentric, wonderful people. . . . For our company, the message is that we're here to produce, sell, and promote artisanal and farmstead cheeses. But that has a big implication and a lot of meaning, because you can't have the farm without the land, you can't sell it without help from a marketing organization, and you can't make better cheese without the University of California extension. We really feel like the other cheeses that are made in this style, and with these same ethics, are as important as the cheese we make."

Cheesemaker, entrepreneur, environmentalist. Sue Conley has many hats, but as she puts it herself, "I'm best at getting the message out. That's really my job." It's a message about delicious, handcrafted food, produced in cooperation with many different environmental and agricultural concerns, and it's a message that can be heard loud and clear, especially in an old barn on a quiet street.

COWGIRL CREAMERY AT TOMALES BAY FOODS
80 Fourth Street
Point Reyes Station, CA 94956
Phone: 415-663-9335
www.cowgirlcreamery.com

Darien Cheese & Fine Foods is my food Mecca. Cross the threshold into this shop in Connecticut and you are transported to a place that does everything right by its food. You can tell just by looking at it. No shrink-wrapped, suffocating cheeses here. Everything is cut to order. Tasting is encouraged—how else to learn which might be your next, can't-live-without-it favorite? I often come in for a wedge or a wheel and walk out with a whole meal. Gorgeous olives glistening in earthenware crocks, salty tapenade to slather on a crusty baguette, prosciutto sliced to order, even handmade chocolates from a local artisan all make for an impromptu dinner party or ready-to-go picnic—and often do.

The proprietors, Ken and Tori Skovron, and their team of knowledgeable and forthright staff not only sell the most flavorful and carefully produced cheeses I have ever found; their philosophy of food production exemplifies the passion, commitment, and joy of the Real Food movement. There's a reverence for the items that they carry. It manifests itself not in a stuffy "worship the cheese" aloofness, but in a dedication to education, to knowing everything they can about each cheese they offer—the breed of the animal providing the milk, the season in which the milk was harvested, the forage the animal was eating. And of course, the background of the producer—how they came to their craft and the special nuance that only that particular cheesemaker can bring to the fromage that they are forging.

Such in-depth knowledge comes from working closely with the producers who ship directly to the store. There is no middleman between Darien Cheese and the farmer, no distributor off-loading surplus wheels. This direct relationship opens up the lines of communication. As Ken describes it, "You get that one-on-one with the farmer, that's the idea. In the process of buying direct you are also discussing the cheeses, the time of the year, making the cheeses better. You don't get that with a distributor." The dialogue dictates what's available at the shop. Ken doesn't just fill out a purchase order and fax it off, as a commercial distributor might. He buys cheeses as they come into season—fresh springtime chèvre is a favorite of mine—or when their makers feel they are ready to leave the creamery.

Although Ken and Tori aren't sticklers about organic certification, producers are screened to make sure that they honor their land and create their cheeses through sustainable means. Ken often visits farmers to reconnect with them and keep up-to-date on their work. He also encourages producers to use traditional practices, such as utilizing unpasteurized milk whenever possible, for both the taste benefits it brings to the product, and the natural enzymatic action that it promotes.

Farmers and cheesemakers benefit from this open communication, but the real winners are the eaters who patronize Darien Cheese. They know that any question asked will be answered with an educated and very candid response—no marketing spin here. And that every item that lines the shelves is best in class—it offers superior flavor and was raised with pride and dignity. What they might not know, however, is that any cheese that requires it is further ripened on site so that selections are offered only at their optimal stage of readiness.

This sort of behind-the-scenes coddling sets Darien Cheese & Fine Foods apart from other retailers who rely on third-party distributors. As Ken explains, "A distributor is really in the business of doing that—distributing product. They're not handlers or ripeners of cheeses. Their warehouses are extremely cold to slow down the ripening of cheeses; they're dry and that's really not a healthy environment for a healthy, living, natural cheese. And then it gets put on a truck in the summertime, in August, and it gets very warm. And so the product gets kind of beat up before it actually gets to the [store]. It's out of the cheesemaker's hands; he can't care for it, nurture it any further. And then the retailer gets it and they're maybe getting it in a condition that cheese shouldn't be sold at. And that's one of the problems with distribution. [When a cheesemaker has] got something that's so special and kind of fragile and unique, it's better that they deal directly [with a retailer] than through a distributor." And it's why eaters, like me, make our pilgrimage to Darien Cheese.

DARIEN CHEESE & FINE FOODS
25-10 Old Kings Highway North
Darien, Connecticut 06820
Phone: 203-655-4344
www.dariencheese.com

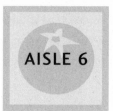

CONVENIENCE FOODS

adore cooking. Always have. A relaxing day for me is an extended stretch in the kitchen, all burners blazing. I cross the finish line when I've run out of ingredients or places in the fridge to store my concoctions. But those days are not every day, and they certainly aren't for everybody. There are days when there is no time, or simply no inclination for anything more than a quick stint at the stove. Work, traffic, bad weather, maybe the early tickle of a cold setting in—we've all been there. You contemplate a run through the drive-thru. Or you come home, drag your starving self to the kitchen, yank open the fridge, and stare blankly at your prospects. What to make for dinner?

INDUSTRIAL AGRICULTURE SNAPSHOT

Companies such as Swanson and Stouffer's would have you believe that the answer is prefab dinner entrées—large portions of coated, sauced, and flavored food chunks, complete with several sides to round out the TV tray. Or perhaps some "just add water to it" concoction from a box or a can. Monikers such as "homestyle" and "healthy choices," and beauty shots of steaming plates can lead you to believe that there's goodness to be had. But cut through the microwaveable film covering and the aroma that rises from your just-nuked repast more closely resembles your dishwater than a delectable feast.

Books such as the *Semi-Homemade* series by Sandra Lee, which show-case recipes that rely on processed foods like Campbell's canned soups, suggest that such products can be the basis for an authentic tasting meal. They reiterate the often-heard mantras that cooking is too time-consuming, or that it requires some bottomless well of knowledge that is too complicated or archaic to plumb.

But that's nonsense. These refrains are just the advertisers talking—sending out an endless string of messages so prolific they hum an undercurrent of white noise through our daily lives. It's this brainwashing—that we're too busy to cook or even to notice what we're eating—that allows them, through finely tuned marketing, to sell nearly worthless ingredients for high prices. To wrap a million-dollar brand around a handful of surplus corn turned into chips and charge us three bucks a bag for it. To replace authentic, delicious ingredients such as butter and cream with cheap imitations like partially hydrogenated vegetable oil and powdered milk and try to distract eaters from noticing.

There is no denying that we are a nation on the go. We have a long to-do list and not a lot of time "to do." No one is more acutely aware of or poised to capitalize on our maxed-out schedules than the food industry. According to a 2002 study by Information Resources, "46 percent of Americans eat most meals away from home or on the go."[1] Marketers prey on the time-crunched with "convenience" foods that are increasingly faster to prepare, quicker to eat, and more portable. "Complete" dinners in a box, pockets, bars, and shakes that offer utensil-free "meals," and snacks in containers designed to fit in your car's cup holders are engineered to keep you eating while you keep moving. Rather than making our life more enjoyable, however, the real advantage of these foods is to conveniently alleviate us of our grocery budget while offering us little benefit—even good taste—in return. Here's a rundown of what you get when you buy some of these convenience items.

The Cheapest, Lowest Quality Ingredients in the Food Industry

Industrially processed foods—convenience food such as snacks, fast food, and heat-and-eat items that are processed by the vat full at a centralized factory—are the garbage dump of the food industry. They are the sponge that absorbs, by the ton, the surplus commodity crops that we don't need but can't seem to stop making too much of, and they are the final destination for scraps from butchering.

It works like this: As discussed on page 125, the price of crops such as corn and soy is so very low that farmers often can't make a living wage growing them. So two things happen—the government pays the farmers subsidies to keep them from going under and the farmers increase production to create some cash flow in increased volume. The result is farmers just barely scraping by and an increasing surplus of grain on the market. If it seems counterintuitive, it is. The taxpayers are funding the growth of a crop of which we already have too much. Who benefits? Big business at every turn. The subsidies grease the engine of industrial agriculture by maintaining demand for the chemicals, equipment, and fossil fuels on which it relies, thus keeping companies that supply them, such as Dow, Monsanto, and Archer Daniels Midland, in business. And the surplus grain provides dirt-cheap raw materials for processors of the snack cakes, corn chips, fast food concoctions, and soda pop that are fast becoming the mainstay of the American diet.

SURPLUS CORN

There's a story meant to educate children about the many uses of corn on the Web site for the National Corn Growers Association.[2] It tells the tale of a little boy baking cupcakes and how these treats couldn't have been made without the grain; there is cornstarch and corn syrup in the cake's decorations, corn sugar in the frosting, and corn oil in the cake. The mom calls them "corny cupcakes," and they aren't just an illustrative example of a promotional piece, they are a metaphor for the ubiquity of surplus crops in the processed food industry.

The dominance of corn in that little guy's recipe is a typical scenario for many convenience foods, which are often nothing more than fantastic combinations of corn in all of its fabricated iterations. Corn refiners would have you believe that finding new uses for corn is clever science being used to put to work an American staple—after all, what could be more homespun and patriotic than employing the heartland's iconic cornstalk? But as discussed in Aisle 4: Grains, Oils, and Sweeteners, agricultural practices that are used to grow our grains on an industrial scale have numerous deleterious effects. They deplete and contaminate our water and soil resources, require tankers of toxic chemicals, are fuel-intensive, and are the breeding ground for GMOs. If anything, we should be looking for ways to grow less grain, not trying to jam it into every edible nook and cranny we can find.

As discussed on page 216, one of the most common uses for corn is the highly refined high fructose corn syrup (HFCS) that sweetens nearly all of the major soft drink brands. It is also used in other products such as jams and baked goods. Beyond HFCS, there are seemingly endless uses for corn—you can find many of them listed on the back of your TV dinner or snack bag. In fact, everything from your dinner at the drive-thru to the snack cake of your coffee break contains its share of the grain, often turning up in places you might not expect. Cornstarch, corn syrup, and corn oil are some of the obvious ones, but modified food starch, xanthan gum, dextrose, and maltodextrin are some other examples of the corn you are eating. Even ingredients such as ascorbic acid and MSG can be derived from corn. Writer Michael Pollan calls chicken nuggets "a most ingenious transubstantiation of corn, from the corn-fed chicken it contains to the bulking and binding agents that hold it together."[3]

Soy is widely regarded among eaters as an extremely healthful food—almost beyond reproach. The halo of wellness that surrounds the bean goes unquestioned, and it is processed into all manner of consumables. But when I walk through the aisles of my local natural foods market and see the "made with soy" label slapped on everything from snack chips and cookies to imitation hamburgers, my suspicion starts to kick in. Are these products really better versions of their non-soy selves or are they just another way that soy growers can off-load their swelling stockpiles? After all, the majority of soy products on the market are genetically modified, which seems a far cry from the back-to-nature image on which soy products such as tofu and tempeh were originally marketed. Ingredients such as textured vegetable protein, soy protein concentrates, and soy protein isolates seem to serve the processed food industry, which relies on them as the building blocks of the food lab, more than anything else.

For vegetarians who avoid meat and vegans who avoid all animal products, or even those with allergies, items like soy burgers and "Notdogs" might be alluring. But processed food is still just that—heavily processed. These convenience items—even those with the glow of a higher consciousness surrounding them—are not good eats.

The most popular use of soy in the U.S. diet, in fact, is the bane of the American diet— it is processed into oil. More than 80 percent of our edible oil comes from soy.[4] In the market, it is simply labeled "vegetable oil."

A large portion of our edible oil is partially hydrogenated—altered to take on a solid texture rather than a liquid. If you are familiar with Crisco in a can, that's partially hydrogenated oil. And this kind of oil is in just about all processed foods. Cookies, crackers, mixes for cakes, biscuits and pancakes, peanut butter, most frozen meals, the majority of margarines and shortenings, microwave popcorn, and snack foods all contain partially hydrogenated fat, and that's bad news.

Now, I am not anti-fat. I love buttery croissants, Southern fried chicken, and even real Mexican food made with genuine lard. Nor am I a nutritionist. But I call such fats natural fats, and, unless you have health reasons to avoid them, they can be part of a vital diet. So bear with me when I say that partially hydrogenated oils are no good. They contain trans fats, which have been linked to high cholesterol, heart disease, and diabetes.[5] An eater doesn't have to be gluttonous to experience the ill effects of trans fats. The processing of these fats, like the processing of high fructose corn syrup discussed on page 217, makes them behave strangely in the human body. They increase bad cholesterol (LDL), decrease good cholesterol (HDL), and have been linked to heart disease and diabetes. In 2003, Health and Human Services Secretary Tommy Thompson said, "Trans fats are bad fats. The less trans fat you and I eat, the healthier we will be."[6]

Such findings have led to an outcry for increased labeling of partially hydrogenated oils on product packaging. Dr. Walter C. Willett, chairman of the nutrition department at the Harvard School of Public Health, says trans fats are much more unhealthful than saturated fats, which are listed on labels.[7] The first to respond with new labeling are the small number of manufacturers who already refuse to use these oils, by stating "no trans fats" or "no partially hydrogenated oils" on their packaging. Although legislation has been passed to require such labeling from all manufacturers, through food industry lobbying it has been postponed, and trans fat labeling is expected to be mandatory in 2006.

Many believe that partially hydrogenated oils, which have become increasingly prevalent since their introduction to the market in the 1970s, are so bad for you that they would never be allowed into the food chain if they were introduced today. So why does the food industry use them? Partially hydrogenated oils are inexpensive and shelf-stable. Indeed, products that contain them, such as Twinkies, seem to have the half-life of their plastic wrappers. This extended stay on the display rack is less costly to the producer, and the use of the oils themselves is much cheaper than the ingredients they are meant to replace, such as butter, but what's in it for the eater?

What the food industry gains in profit, we lose in taste. You can really tell the difference. Amanda Hesser, describing the taste of partially hydrogenated oil as "grainy and flabby," in the *New York Times*, says it leaves "a coating of grease on [her] tongue."[8] Compare pure creamery butter, the traditional fat in many baked goods, to partially hydrogenated oil, which is the industry standard in commercial confections. The buttery goodness of a home-baked cookie, the luscious frosting on that chocolate cake at your favorite restaurant—that's butter. The coated feeling you get on your tongue from eating cookies from a box, the gritty, super-sweet frosting on that cellophane-wrapped cupcake—that's partially hydrogenated vegetable oil.

CHEAP MEAT

Cheap ingredients are not limited to surplus crops like corn and soy. There's a reason why you don't see a lot of filet mignon in TV dinners. The finest, freshest cuts of meat are reserved for preparations where their quality will be noticed and appreciated—like a run under the broiler at your favorite restaurant or showcased by your kitchen handiwork at home. Items that are destined to be ground, injected, cooked, frozen, shipped, stored, and reheated again needn't hold a pedigree. At the least, meats that are in the majority of convenience items are the cutting scraps from better cuts—like the little flap of meat on the back of a chicken breast or the better half of a bruised thigh that gets turned into a breaded strip, for example. At the worst, they are the by-products of meat processing—such as the paste-like extrusion that is extracted from a butchered carcass and is the "beef" in the majority of all-beef hot dogs. This kind of meat is of such low quality that it has been brought under fire as one of the leading vectors for transmission of mad cow disease to humans.

It's Expensive

PAYING FOR SCIENCE

If you're not paying for the quality of the ingredients, then what are you paying for? Well, the processing, for one. It takes a lot of science to figure out how to make chicken salad out of chicken feathers, so to speak. Food science is funded by agribusiness, and agribusiness is funded by you each time you buy these products.

PAYING FOR ADVERTISING

When you buy processed food, a substantial portion of your grocery dollar goes to the advertising and marketing that entices you to put it in your cart. In her enlightening book, *Food Politics,* Marion Nestle observes, "In total, food companies spent more than $33 billion annually at the turn of the century to advertise and promote their products to the public."[9] And the message is working. Jeremy J. Fingerman, president of the United States soup division of Campbell Soup in Camden, New Jersey, says his company has estimated that the market for convenience foods is growing by 14 to 16 percent a year.[10]

PAYING FOR CONVENIENCE

Those eaters aren't buying the food because it is delicious. They're buying it because they've been convinced that the convenience is worth the price. "Food companies used to focus on taste, taste, taste, but now you see convenience as almost—if not as—important," said John McMillin, a food industry analyst at the Prudential Equity Group in New York.[11] According to Information Resources, Inc., a market research firm in Chicago, shoppers are willing to pay two to three times more per serving for the same food if it is presented in an easier-to-consume way.[12] That's a lot to pay for the luxury of not using utensils or being denied the joy of a home-cooked meal.

Loss of Culture

This is not to say that we don't all get caught now and again with more hunger than time. But when wolfing down a burger in the car becomes your regular lunch routine, your idea of a leisurely meal is to reheat your frozen entrée in the oven instead of the microwave, and your kids think that potato chips count as a vegetable, you might want to rethink your strategy. Meals are more than a way to fill your belly; they can be an oasis in a hectic schedule, a planned time, each day, to sit, chat, and reflect on the day.

Enjoying our meals rather than consuming them is a concept that might be becoming foreign to us in this country. Although McDonald's is spreading like a plague across the globe, the addiction to the wider category of convenience foods—microwaveable dinners, grab-and-go snacks—is uniquely American. "[Convenience food] is definitely a growing trend in the United States," Lynn Dornblaser, editor of the *Global New Product Database,* created by the Mintel International Group, a market research firm, said, but not in Europe or Latin America because "it's not in their culture to eat on the run."[13]

Our treatment of food as fuel—and nothing more—is chipping away at our heritage. Recipes that used to get passed down from generation to generation are now being displaced by the heat-and-eat, "home-cooked" dinner entrée. Traveling abroad, you can dine like a king on the peasant food—the staple dishes—of other nations. The slow cooked stew, feijoada, in Brazil. Rice and beans in Mexico. Pot-au-feu in France. These are all affordable dishes that cooks have made for generations with simple ingredients they have on hand. We are trading in the waft of the stew pot for the high-toned beep of the microwave.

Edges Out the Small Farmer

Eaters are not the only ones who lose out in the processed food game— small farmers lose their edge in this arena, as well. The overhead—the machinery, staff, and advertising—that it takes to get a processed product to a profitable stage requires the kind of capital investment that often only a large entity can float. You might think that food processing creates a market for farmers—a place to sell their goods—but more often than not, large processors can only afford to deal with large growers and producers who can guarantee huge shipments of the same ingredient. For example, it takes the milk from 16,000 cows to supply Red Baron pizza, the largest manufacturer of frozen mini-pizzas, with its supply of cheese topping every day.[14]

Bad for the Environment

PROMOTES MONOCULTURE

All this leads to one of the biggest environmental issues associated with processed food—monoculture. As discussed throughout the book, monoculturing, the intensive growing of only one species over a large area or in a crowded population, leaves the plant or animal vulnerable to disease and stresses the surrounding environment. Processed food, because it demands huge amounts of identical product, promotes the development of monocultures.

Take potatoes, for example. Worldwide, there are more than five thousand varieties of potatoes.[15] The varieties are extremely diverse: Some taste so buttery you'd swear they were half dairy, some are starchy and bland. They come in all shapes and sizes, from small and round to long and thin, and are quite colorful—white, yellow, red, blue, even purple. Yet more than half the world's potato acreage is now planted with one variety of potato: the Russet Burbank used by McDonald's.[16] It is this potato alone that will produce the long, thin shoestrings that sit up so nicely in the red cartons used by the golden arches worldwide.[17]

Even if fast food restaurants and other convenience food conglomerates switched to an all-organic menu tomorrow, they would still be sucking the life out of our farms by imposing demand for raw materials so uniform they can only be produced in monoculture environments. This sameness also extends to a shift in our taste buds. After a lifetime of eating processed foods—perfectly shaped, uniform french fries, round bacon on our breakfast sandwiches—the real, flavorful, natural food starts to look and taste obscure. We as eaters start to regard the purple potatoes of the world as wrong because they look foreign, when in fact it is the purple variety that is the more flavorful, more "natural," than the Russet Burbank.

INCREASED PESTICIDE USE

The quest for similarity in processed food also can lead to an increased use of agricultural chemicals. Take those same fast food fries, for example. As Michael Pollan describes in *The Botany of Desire: A Plant's Eye View of the World,* some of the most deadly toxins used on potato farms are implemented for purely cosmetic reasons—so that our fries won't have brown spots on them.[18] If we could let go of the need for a perfectly golden fry, we could eliminate the use of such poisons.

Source of GMOs

For a time, McDonald's sought to extend the model of perfection even further by experimenting with a genetically modified potato. Fortunately, eaters got wind of the plan and negative consumer reaction stopped the use of the GMO spuds in its tracks.

However, GMOs still dominate the processed food market. Surplus soy and corn crops are currently the major sources of genetically modified ingredients in our diet. So it follows that processed food, which is largely made up of these products, is high in GMO content. Up to 60 percent of processed foods in the United States have some GMO ingredient.[19]

Large-Plant Processing Is More Vulnerable

The large scale on which food processing profitability relies makes us vulnerable to food-borne illness. Listeria may be a word that rings a bell. It is a food-borne bacteria that is most associated with processed meats such as the roast beef and turkey you buy at the deli. While any food can carry listeria, cooking kills the bacteria. That is why deli meat, which is usually eaten uncooked, is often the culprit of listeriosis, the sickness that develops from ingesting the pathogens. Listeriosis causes flu-like symptoms that are often misdiagnosed, making it hard to determine the rate of contamination in our food supply. But the numbers are so high that pregnant women and those with compromised immune systems are advised to avoid foods such as lunch meats, which may be contaminated, completely.

Processed Food Is Loaded with Preservatives

Salt, sugar, nitrites, and nitrates are flavor enhancers and preservatives used in much food processing. Not to argue the health implications of consuming such agents, but I do have friends who complain of hot dog headaches from the nitrites and nitrates commonly found in those items. And I'm pretty sure that everyone would agree that salt and sugar are not ingredients that one should be enjoying by the can or bag full. It's easy, though, to load up on these ingredients without even realizing it when you are eating a lot of processed food. They act as preservatives, extending shelf life and preserving the color of food that has to hang around for extended periods. They also act as a flavor enhancer for the rather bland ingredients that are used in manufactured food. If you are avoiding them, cutting out processed food is a great way to do it. If you are doing your own cooking, you have total control over the ingredients.

Transportation and Production Are Fuel Intensive

Processed food is incredibly energy intensive. Think about it. If you buy some vegetables from the farmers' market, bring them home, and make a stir-fry, you have spent the gas in your car to get them; the rest is mostly manual labor—the farmer's work, your chopping. Maybe a few pennies spent on whatever fuel heats your stove, but that's it. Now, if you pick up a bag of frozen stir-fry dinner, you've started this chain reaction: Each vegetable has been grown on a monoculture farm where it is planted, raised, and harvested by large gas-guzzling machines—fuel for farming. Because the variety of veggies in the bag was harvested at different places, it all had to be transported to a central processing plant—fuel for transport. There the vegetables were washed, chopped, and packaged mechanically by a factory that requires a mini–power plant to run it—fuel for processing. The vegetables are then packaged, stored, transported, and displayed all under constant refrigeration to maintain their frozen state (the freezers that house frozen foods for distribution can be the size of an office building[20])—fuel for cooling and storage. Then the bag finally makes it to your house, where it takes up real estate in your freezer—more fuel for storage—until you put it on your dinner plate.

Packaging Waste

Then you throw out the bag, adding to the landfill!

Worst for the Kids

Processed food might be a bad food choice for adult eaters, but it is absolutely wrecking our kids. They might beg for chicken nuggets and pine for another trip through the drive-thru, but this route is a dead-end street. What kids need is not the quick fix, but a connection to food that nourishes them and that will inform their eating decisions as they grow older.

Advertisers know the importance of building eating patterns at a young age. That's why McDonald's is one of the largest purveyors of toys in the nation.[21] Enticing kids with toys to eat at their establishment is only one way to incite what marketers call the nag factor—the persuasiveness of a tiny voice, particularly when used in repetitive fashion, in influencing the household's dinner choices. Other methods of seduction include children's characters emblazoned on the front of food cartons and drink packages, foods artificially colored into neon shades to attract attention, and even pressed into shapes of their favorite idols.

Everywhere they turn, kids are bombarded by advertising for processed food. I expected to see such marketing in the media, but was shocked the first time I went toy shopping for my little girl. She loves to cook, so I wanted to get her her own "kitchen." I was horrified to find that the cook sets were branded by fast food chains—complete with fry-o-lators and burger flippers. A children's clothing line at Wal-Mart is sponsored by McDonald's, and bears the brand's logo. I've even seen baby bottles with sugary beverage logos on them.

The advertising strategy is working, but with horrendous results. According to a study reported in *Pediatrics* magazine, "Every day, nearly one-third of U.S. children aged 4 to 19 eat fast food, which likely packs on about 6 extra pounds per child a year and increases the risk of obesity."[22] Eating processed food such as fast food, soft drinks, and snacks is being blamed for other children's health issues, such as type two diabetes, which was previously only seen in adults. It is feared that due to the current imbalance of lack of exercise and increased consumption of processed foods this generation of children will be the first to die before their parents.[23]

One would think—at least I did—that schools would play some role in teaching kids about good nutrition. In fact, the opposite is often true. School districts accept money, through a variety of revenue streams, from the processed food industry. School districts permit Channel One, the television network for schools, to broadcast two minutes a day of commercials by McDonald's, Hershey, PepsiCo, Coca-Cola, Frito-Lay, and the like.[24] Some schools sell "pouring rights" to cola bottlers—granting exclusive vending rights in exchange for monetary kickbacks. Schools also can sign vending contracts, from which they receive part of the profits, for high-fat, high-calorie, high-sugar candy, cookies, chips, and ice cream. Fundraising drives collect money by selling more junk food.[25] According to the Centers for Disease Control, vending machines provide money for 98 percent of public high schools, 74 percent of middle schools, and 43 percent of elementary schools.[26]

The lunch programs themselves offer no information about a sustainable diet. My kids aren't in school yet, but every once in a while I'll glance at the local newspaper's listing of the weekly menu for the area's school lunch program. Invariably it is the same, just rearranged on various days, to include pizza, chicken nuggets, patty melts, tacos, and the mysterious "chuck wagon." What kind of lesson is this? A sad fact of our scholastic history is that school cafeterias aren't even equipped any longer to prepare fresh food. There are no cooking utensils, no pans, no knives, not a chopping board in sight. School cafeterias are only prepared to reheat the substandard government subsidized fare that is shipped to them in bulk. (Read the Profile of the Ross School on page 207 where eating Real Food is part of the curriculum.)

Some would argue that that's the kind of food kids want. But I think adults are often very far off base when it comes to guessing what kids desire. In a 1999 study conducted by Ellen Galinsky, President of the Families and Work Institute in New York, parents and their children ages eight through eighteen were asked what they thought children would most remember about this period in their lives. Galinsky said, "When I asked parents, they would often guess the big moments. The family vacation. The special event. Kids would talk about everyday family rituals."[27]

The fondest memories are not built on the one hundred and first burger that you grabbed on the go, but on the shared familial activity of preparing food together. Of talking at the end of the day over a delicious meal. It doesn't have to be fancy—just turn off the TV and break some bread.

Nancé's Crockpot Pot Roast

My mom worked full-time when I was a kid. This rich, delicious roast—which practically cooks itself—is a little trick she taught me for getting dinner on the table no matter how busy your day.

For the Roast
2 tablespoons olive oil
One 4-pound chuck roast or bottom-round roast
½ bottle dry red wine

1 bay leaf
1 teaspoon dried thyme
Salt and freshly ground black pepper
2 carrots, roughly chopped
1 medium tomato, halved
1 head garlic, cloves peeled and separated
1 celery stalk, halved

For the Gravy
Liquid from the roast
2 tablespoons all-purpose flour
2 tablespoons unsalted butter, softened
Salt and freshly ground black pepper

To make the roast: Heat the oil in a medium skillet over medium heat. Add the roast and sear on all sides until brown all over, about 5 minutes per side. Put the roast in a crockpot and turn on Low. Add the remaining ingredients in the order listed and cover the pot. Cook for 8 hours. Remove the roast from the pot, strain the liquid, and discard the solids.

To make the gravy: Place the liquid from the roast in a small saucepan or saucier over medium-high heat. Bring to a boil and reduce the liquid by half to strengthen the flavor. The flavor should be slightly more assertive than desired. While the sauce is reducing, combine the flour and butter in a small dish using a fork until completely blended to make beurre marnier or raw roux. Add roux in small amounts to the liquid, whisking with each addition, until the sauce is desired thickness. Season with salt and pepper to taste. Serve with the roast.

Serves 4 to 6

REVIVING REAL FOOD

Use these tips so you don't shortchange your taste buds when you're short on time.

Avoid Partially Hydrogenated Oils

Look for snacks that don't contain partially hydrogenated oils. Chips made from potatoes, oil, and salt, and baked (organic, small-batch) tortilla chips are a good start.

Buy Organic

Organic processed food does offer a better option to conventional products in that it will lower your exposure to chemical residues. However, all manufactured food, even organic, carries with it a similar burden of the process. You are still paying for the science to develop such products, the marketing and advertising to make you aware of them, and the fuel costs involved in manufacturing, shipment, and storage. And even organic foods often contain binders and fillers, additives and preservatives, that are the nature of the processing beast—that keep sauces from separating, your tomato sauce tomato-red, and your cookies from crumbling. When you buy processed food, any processed food, you are paying for all of these things.

Unlike whole foods, which are either organic or not (see individual chapters for more information), there are four levels of labeling in packaged foods that have more than one ingredient.

100% ORGANIC
Everything in the package must be certified organic—that is, grown and processed without traditional agriculture chemicals, artificial hormones,

or antibiotics. Such items can say 100 percent organic on the label, can bear the USDA Organic seal (see below), and must list the certifying agent.

ORGANIC

Ninety-five percent of the contents must be certified organic. The product may not contain added sulfites. The product may be called organic, can bear the USDA seal, and must list the certifying agent.

MADE WITH ORGANIC

Seventy-five to ninety-four percent of the contents must be certified organic. The product may list such ingredients on the front panel of the packaging. The product must identify the certifying agent. It cannot use the USDA Organic seal.

LISTED ORGANIC INGREDIENTS

Products that contain fewer than 75 percent organic ingredients may list those ingredients as organic in the ingredients list (for example: flour, sugar, organic carrots). The word "organic" may not appear on the front panel of the packaging, the USDA Organic seal cannot be used, and the certifying agents needn't be listed.

Support Your Local Eateries

Pass by the national fast food chain and head to the local deli, pizza parlor, Chinese takeout, or taco stand. You'll be supporting a small, perhaps family business and keeping your food dollars in your community. And, unlike a national chain, you have direct access to the operation's decision maker, the owner, so your opinions about the food get heard.

Look for Smaller "Readable" Brands

Okay, so if you haven't noticed, I'm not big on processed foods. But I'd be lying if I said there isn't a box or two in my pantry of "emergency meals." For these I rely on small brands that offer, at the very least, an ingredient list that I can read. If I can't pronounce it, I don't buy it. But a jar of tomato sauce full of ingredients I could actually find in my pantry and not the science lab, or that isn't loaded with enough sugar to qualify as a dessert is okay to have rattling around on the back of the shelf—anything to avoid the drive-thru.

Eat Real Fruit

Fruit-flavored treats are not the same as fruits. Fruit roll-ups and leathers can be mostly sugar. Opt for whole fruits instead. And be as selective with any frozen fruit as you would with fresh produce. They're both subject to the same issues of sustainability—such as toxic chemical applications during and after growing—with frozen items having the added ecological burdens of transportation and electricity usage required to maintain their frozen state.

Beware "100% Beef"

Beef can be anything that comes from a cow. It does not necessarily mean muscle cuts.

Involve Your Kids

Kitchens are great places for kids—they're like in-house science labs that can turn a bowl full of raw eggs and flour into a birthday cake. Any kid can get involved—two-year-olds make great tomato squishers. Older kids can chop mushrooms and other soft ingredients with their own plastic knife. "Measuring" and "mixing" bowls of dried beans is fair play for any kid. Involve your kids in the cooking and they are more likely to try what's on their plate.

Kids may not be the neatest planters, but they may very well be the most enthusiastic, according to Randy Woodard, the Greenhouse Manager at Cabbage Hill Farm in Mount Kisco, New York, who works with kids in the field. "Basically you've got certain things that didn't germinate and they're all going every which way, but the kids are loving it," he explains. "They take ownership. They can't wait to pick it and wash and eat it up. It's super." Even if you don't have a green thumb, a tomato or pepper plant in a pot or some herbs on the windowsill are enough to show how things grow.

Keep your kids in touch with where their food comes from. Visit a farm one weekend or, better yet, join a CSA, or develop a farmers' market habit where the kids can get in tune with the rhythm of the seasons.

Don't rely on the school to feed your children well. Send them off with the old-fashioned brown-bagged lunch and know what they are eating.

Keep a Well-Stocked Pantry

Nothing says convenience like having a library of delicious ingredients at your fingertips. I can remember walking through my Granny Toni's pantry. It was like perusing a little market. Shelves were lined with mason jars of peaches from her trees, tomatoes from her vines, pickles that she made out of the cucumbers that she grew. Then there were jars of prepared things, too. Homemade marinara sauce, jams and preserves from the fruit trees. Herbs hung from the ceiling beams to dry. Every night before dinner she would send me down there to "shop" for the ingredients she needed for her dishes.

While you might not have the penchant for "putting by" that my Granny did, maintaining a well-stocked pantry—a collection of frozen, canned, and dried items that you keep on hand—can be your emergency kit when you haven't made it to the market, are short on time, or need a backdrop for the disparate selections of ingredients that you picked up at the farmers' market. Most of the items are things that I "process" myself—such as berries, peppers, and herbs that I keep on hand in the freezer. Others are stocks, sauces, and bases that are the building blocks of some hearty dishes. Canned tomatoes and dried wild mushrooms allow me to access these seasonal flavors all year long. And of course, no pantry would be complete without a good selection of high-quality organic dried spices. Here are some pointers on putting your pantry together.

First and Foremost, Stay Seasonal

Shelf-stable items are never going to have the same bright flavors and textures as those fresh out of the garden. So make your selections carefully. Only use these backup ingredients in small quantities when you can't get fresh, or when your supply of "put by" items runs out. A package of frozen peas is fine to dump into a stew for a little color boost, but wait for spring when fresh ones are available to give them the spotlight. Use them in dishes that will mask their deficiencies rather than pointing up their shortcomings. You'd never use canned tomatoes in a salsa where the soft texture of the fruit would bring down the dish, but in a slow-cooked tomato sauce, there's nothing better.

Limit Residues, Additives, and Preservatives

It's important to be aware of any chemical residues in your pantry items. In some cases, even more so than in your fresh foods, as processing methods such as drying may intensify any toxins that were present in the food in its natural state. Buy organic when you can to cut down on the use of chemical inputs at the farm level and the residues in the things you eat.

And, because foods that you keep in your pantry are meant to be stored, they are inclined to have additives and preservatives in them to extend their shelf life. Opt for frozen items over canned, which typically contain preservatives and high amounts of salt to extend their shelf life, maintain their color, and to—futilely in my opinion—retain their texture. If you are storing dried items, seek out those without sulfur—an unnecessary additive used to preserve color.

Limit Resource Useage

Frozen and canned items require a lot of resources to get from field to table. Often this overhead is too large of a hurdle for a small producer to overcome, so canned and frozen items often become the domain of large conglomerates that can realize economies of scale. So keep your supply of store-bought preserved produce low. When buying frozen items, avoid vegetable medleys, succotash, and other combos that require additional shipping from their individual points of origin to be processed. Opt for single-ingredient items and mix them yourself at home.

Because they are lightweight to ship and require no refrigeration, dried foods are a less resource-intensive option than canned or frozen foods. Dried fruits, rehydrated in some hot water, juice, or wine can add some tang to stuffings, salads, and desserts. Dried mushrooms are a great component of hearty dishes such as risottos. Opt for dried tomatoes and rehydrate them in hot water rather than buying them packed in oil to cut down on extra shipping weight.

Wild Mushroom Risotto

Low and slow is the secret to good risotto. You have to be patient with this dish—it should take about 45 minutes from start to finish, but the results are delicious and you can use the leftovers for another great meal, Risotto Cakes (recipe follows), for lunch or dinner the next day.

- 1 ounce dried wild mushrooms such as morels or chanterelles
- ¼ cup plus 2 tablespoons olive oil
- ½ pound assorted fresh mushrooms such as portobello or shiitake, sliced
- 1 shallot, finely diced
- Salt and freshly ground black pepper
- 1 pound arborio rice
- 1 teaspoon dried thyme
- 1 cup dry white wine
- 8 cups hot chicken stock, preferably homemade (see recipe, page 79)
- 4 ounces Parmigiano Reggiano cheese, grated
- ¼ cup chopped fresh parsley

Rehydrate the mushrooms: Place the dried mushrooms in a small heatproof bowl, and pour 2 cups boiling water over them. Cover and set aside to steep for at least 30 minutes. Remove the rehydrated mushrooms from liquid, reserving the liquid. Finely chop the mushrooms. Strain the mushroom liquid through a coffee filter to capture any grit and set aside.

Make the risotto: Heat 2 tablespoons of the oil in a heavy-bottomed Dutch oven over medium-high heat. Add the fresh mushrooms and sauté until they begin to color—they will give off their liquid and then begin to turn golden. Add the shallot and salt and pepper to taste and sauté 1 to 3 minutes, until tender. Add the remaining ¼ cup oil and the rice to the pot and sauté the rice until the grains turn pearly and opaque, 3 to 5 minutes. Add the thyme and wine. Reduce the heat to medium-low and simmer, stirring constantly, until the wine is absorbed. Add the reserved mushroom liquid and rehydrated mushrooms to the rice and stir until the liquid is absorbed. Add hot stock, 1 cup at a time, stirring constantly and waiting until the liquid is nearly absorbed and the rice threatens to stick to the pan bottom before adding the next cup. Continue adding stock in this manner until the rice is tender and the risotto has a creamy consistency, about 35 minutes. Remove from the heat. Add half of the grated cheese, all of the parsley, and salt and pepper to taste. Pass the remaining cheese to sprinkle on each serving.

Serves 4, with leftovers

Risotto Cakes

Serve over a green salad for lunch or a light dinner. You can also serve them topped with marinara sauce (see recipe, page 82).

½ cup olive oil
Leftovers from Wild Mushroom Risotto (page 201), chilled
1 cup fresh breadcrumbs
1 cup freshly grated Parmesan cheese
1 egg, slightly beaten

Heat the oil in a heavy-bottomed skillet over medium high heat. While the oil is heating, form the leftover risotto into palm-size patties (chilled risotto will hold its shape). Combine the breadcrumbs and cheese in a shallow dish. Pour the egg into a separate shallow dish. Dip the patties,

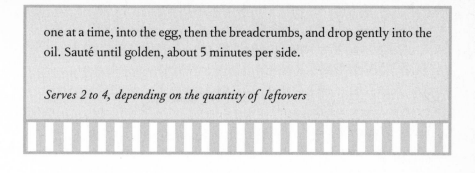
Keep a Library of Stocks and Bases

I keep a variety of stocks in quart-sized freezer bags in the deep freeze. I use the stock in everything—soups, stews, rice dishes, or ladled into the skillet in which I've just browned a steak or some chicken for a quick pan sauce. You don't have to buy ingredients to make stock, just use chef Jacques Pepin's trick. Keep an empty milk carton on the door of your freezer. Put meat scraps and the peels and ends of things like onions, carrots, and celery in there as you produce them. Any vegetable that is not too strong, like cabbage or broccoli are, is fine. When the carton is full, peel away the container and dump the entire contents in a pot of water to cover,

Vegetable Stock

Sautéing the vegetables first brings a richness to this stock and keeps it from tasting too green or raw.

- 2 tablespoons organic canola oil
- 1 quart vegetable trimmings (such as onion tops, garlic skins, carrot shavings, or parsley stems—avoid any strongly flavored vegetables such as broccoli or cabbage)

1 bouquet garni (bay leaf, sprigs of thyme and parsley, and 6 pepper-corns, tied in a knot of cheesecloth or enclosed in a tea ball) (optional)

Heat the oil in a large Dutch oven or stockpot over medium heat. Add the vegetable trimmings and sauté until they begin to color, about 15 minutes. Add 2 quarts cold water and the bouquet garni, if using, and bring to a simmer. Reduce the heat to low and simmer for 1 hour. Cool, strain, and refrigerate until completely chilled. Remove any fat from the top of the chilled stock. Divide the stock into freezer bags and freeze until ready to use.

Makes one quart

simmer for two to three hours, then strain. You'll be rewarded with a beautiful stock.

Store intensely flavored items like pestos and caramelized onions in ice cube trays. I melt one or two of the pesto cubes on top of a piece of grilled fish or steak, or throw them in a bowl of noodles or rice, add a handful of cheese, a few leaves of spinach or arugula, toss, and dinner is served.

Easy Pesto

Make this vibrant pesto in the summertime when basil is threatening to overtake your garden or can be found in large bouquets in the farmers' market. Don't hesitate to double the recipe if you find yourself with a wealth of the fresh herb on hand.

I use a handheld blender to whip this up quickly without creating too much washing-up work. You can also use a blender or food processor—just combine the first four ingredients, give it a whir, then add the basil and puree—but you'll need to mince the garlic before adding it to the appliance or it won't be adequately pulverized. You can freeze the pureed pesto in an ice cube tray and store the frozen cubes in a Ziploc bag in the freezer until ready to use.

   2 garlic cloves (minced if using a blender or food processor)
   ½ cup olive oil
   ½ cup pine nuts (also called pignoli nuts)
   1 cup freshly grated Parmesan cheese (preferably Parmigiano Reggiano)
   1 cup firmly packed fresh basil leaves
   Salt and freshly ground black pepper

Place the garlic and oil in a medium bowl. Puree with a handheld blender to mince the garlic. Add the pine nuts and cheese and puree until smooth. Add the basil and puree again until uniformly green. Add salt and pepper to taste. Use as a topping for pasta, a sandwich spread, or as a flavoring agent for rice, or whir a frozen cube of pesto with ½ cup olive oil and 2 tablespoons red wine vinegar for a quick salad dressing or marinade for poultry.

Makes just over 2 cups

MMMMM BEANS

I love long-cooked beans. I find those in the can to be too mushy, and the liquid that they are canned in is unappetizing to me. I always make a double batch of home-cooked beans and freeze some for later. If you put a little of the cooking liquid in their freezer container, they can be the base for a quick bean soup or can be sautéed in a whopping amount of garlic (I use one head of garlic per quart of beans) for great refried beans or for a quick meal.

Greens and Beans on Toast

This recipe is a throwback to my bachelorette days, but it's a family favorite now.

2 tablespoons olive oil
1 small onion, finely diced
2 cloves garlic, minced
1 bunch greens, such as spinach, chard, or kale, roughly chopped
1 cup Slow-Cooked White Beans (see recipe, page 74)
Salt and freshly ground black pepper
4 baguette slices, cut on the diagonal (the bread may be slightly stale or frozen)
High-quality olive oil, for drizzling
¼ cup grated Parmesan cheese

Heat the oil in a medium sauté pan over medium heat. Add the onion and sauté until translucent, 5 to 7 minutes. Add the garlic and sauté until fragrant, 1 minute. Add the greens and sauté until wilted. Add the beans and cook until heated through. Season with salt and pepper to taste. While the beans are heating, toast the bread until golden on both sides and crisp throughout. Place 2 slices of toast on each of 2 plates. Top each serving with half of the greens and beans mixture. Drizzle with the high-quality olive oil, sprinkle with cheese, and serve.

Serves 2

Try Your Hand at the Can

During the summer months when farmstands are overflowing with ripe tomatoes, corn is at its sweetest, and your office mate overplanted his zucchini patch, take a stab at "putting by." Can up the bounty and enjoy it all winter. Plus, you'll have shelves stocked with those adorable mason jars.

FREEZE A TASTE OF SUMMER

Not up for canning? Your freezer can become a savings bank of fresh flavors if you snap up fruits and vegetables at their peak and put them in the freezer for another day. Blanch items like peaches and tomatoes to remove skins, then seal in quart-sized zipper bags (that you can rinse and reuse) and freeze. Sear or broil peppers until their skins char, close them up in a sealed container or bag for five minutes, then slip off skins and freeze the smoky roasted pepper flesh. Rinse, dry, and freeze berries in a single layer on a cookie sheet, then transfer to bags. Freeze washed herbs covered with water or pureed in oil in ice cube trays, then transfer to bags when solid.

MAKE YOUR OWN TV DINNERS

The next time you cook dinner, make extra and freeze it in individual portions for a quick meal anytime.

PROFILE: THE ROSS SCHOOL

The lunchroom at the Ross School in East Hampton, New York, is called "the Café," not the cafeteria, and it's an important distinction. "Cafeteria" conjures up food fights, a quick ten minutes between classes surrounded by the noise of many children chattering and wolfing down mystery meat. A café, on the other hand, is a place to enjoy food, a place to relax, a place for all ages. And that's exactly what the Ross School Café is. The large room, which reflects the mix of Eastern and Western influences that are central to the school's philosophy—the decor is Asian and the students don slippers before entering—does not feel at all like a typical school eatery. "You go in here, and you know, we do 1,300 meals a day, 200,000 meals a year, but you go in here and it feels like a restaurant," says Ann Cooper, former Executive Chef and Director of Wellness and Nutrition at the school. "And it's a little loud, but it feels like a loud restaurant—a loud, busy, happening place. It certainly doesn't sound like a cafeteria. You close your eyes, you'd be hard-pressed to know it was kids, not adults. . . . It's about dining as opposed to fueling. That's one of the things we talk to the kids a lot about."

Talking about food is key to the success of the Ross School, where kids not only eat their vegetables; they pile them high on their plates. The school places great importance on learning how to make better food choices. "If we're not teaching kids about food, then who is? Coke and McDonald's are," says Ann. Such education is imperative, she believes, if the younger generation is going to be able to turn the tide of industrial food production. "Now we've got a generation of children who thinks that safe, healthy food is something you stick your arm out a window for, and somebody—you have no idea who they are or the last time they washed their hands—hands you a bag and you sit there and eat it, in the car. That's become dining. We've got to stop."

There is no fast food at the Ross School. "We give our kids forty minutes for lunch here, where you know most public schools are twenty or thirty [minutes long]. You know, if you want someone to dine, you've got to give them time." There are also no vending machines. Instead, bowls of seasonal fruit are on offer throughout every school building on the wooded campus. "What we do is put really good food out. It's fresh, it's seasonal. There are no tricks, it's very recognizable for the most part." In addition to gourmet pizza just turned out of a wood-burning stove and a salad bar brimming with seasonal and often local fruits and veggies—both of which are everyday staples—there are several different menu options on offer that cover all of the dietary idiosyncrasies—vegetarian, kosher, vegan—of a varied student body. The day I visited, I saw many students helping themselves to a little of everything, including many foods that some people might think a kid would never consider—tofu in an authentic Mexican mole sauce, for instance.

Food education at the Ross School goes beyond the one-size-fits-all, "it's good for you" message that falls on the deaf ears of kids that aren't engaged in their food choices. It's put into the context of their lives—athletes are encouraged to bank energy for sports through their food choices, for example. A roving nutritionist passes through the Café as kids eat and talks to the students about what's on their plate at that instant. Kids get their hands dirty during practical lessons in the fields of neighboring farms. A garden outside of the Café reminds everyone that, as Ann puts it, "Food comes from dirt, not out of a plastic package."

The food is given respect and the kids are, too. Food is not "dumbed down" for them—the Café serves up grilled chicken paillards, for example, vs. breaded chicken dinosaur shapes. "[Kids] are just younger people. And we've got to stop treating them like they're something else. They're not. They're not from Mars. . . . You know, a lot is garnered from respect."

So here's what happens when you give kids a lot of information about their food, time to enjoy it, and the respect to make intelligent choices. They eat healthy and sustainable food. "The Café should be a classroom," Ann says. "If you want to be successful, you've got to put just as much importance on the Café as math, English, or science. And I think all the geometry in the world is not going to save you if you can't eat well and don't have good health. What good is trigonometry if you die at forty? . . . We really have to think about that and make wellness and nutrition a real core value of everybody's lives."

THE ROSS SCHOOL
18 Goodfriend Drive
East Hampton, New York 11937
Phone: 631-329-5245
www.ross.org

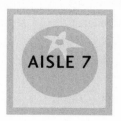

AISLE 7

BEVERAGES

I t's part and parcel of the gracious greeting. Whether it's a meeting in your office ("Can I get you something?"), a trip to the local diner ("Coffee?"), or a belly-up to the bar ("Whattayahavin?"), the offering of a beverage is a vestige of hospitality that survives in even the coarsest social situation. It was a reward in ancient times to the weary traveler who had undoubtedly gone through greater travails than crosstown traffic to see you. And today the tradition remains the verbal equivalent of dusting off the welcome mat. Meeting a friend for coffee or sharing some cool lemonade on the porch swing turns a cup of joe or some flavored water into a social event.

From the products from which they are made, the methods of marketing and distribution that bring them to you, to the quality of the final product, what you choose to drink has greater impact than slaking your thirst. When you pick up that cup of java, pop the top off of your sports-size water bottle, or pour your kid a sippy cup full of Florida's finest, you are validating all of the choices that were made to bring that sip to your lips.

This chapter is structured a little differently from the others; it's really four mini-chapters, one on each type of drink—coffee and tea, water, juice, and soft drinks. Each gives some background on that drink category, followed by some strategies for making choices in the marketplace.

Coffee and Tea

You may not be thinking much about it as you hazily reach for your morning cup of wake-up, but that eight-ounce mug of steaming goodness can do a lot of good in the world. It can guarantee a decent wage for a farmer so he doesn't have to resort to planting less-than-legal crops to make ends meet. It can support the habits of migratory birds so they don't go extinct. It can send a farmer's kid—first in the family to go—to school every day. Or not. Here's how.

INDUSTRIAL AGRICULTURE SNAPSHOT

It may be hard to believe as you shell out five dollars for a mocha latte, but for most of the world's farmers, growing coffee beans is not a lucrative business. The majority of the profit goes to the many middlemen who handle the beans before they make their way into the brew you hold in your hand. The wholesalers and buyers, roasters, distributors, the marketers, the shop owners, even that inattentive kid behind the counter, all get a bigger piece of the pie than the farmer who grows the crop. According to Rodney North, in the book *Sustainable Cuisine White Papers*, the typical coffee farmer has only a small plot of five acres or fewer, is dependent on one local buyer, has no access to information about the market or sustainable practices, has no access to financing, and often becomes indebted to the local buyer.[1] It's the picture of repression.

Added to which, in fewer than twenty years the price of coffee has fallen through the floor. Wholesale coffee on world markets now sells for about 55 cents a pound, compared with $1.20 in the 1980s.[2] There are a number of factors that have contributed to this shift in the market, but many see the 1989 exit of the United States from the International Coffee Organization (ICO), which stabilized worldwide prices through a regimen of production quotas, as its catalyst. After the pullout, Brazil increased production and Vietnam flooded the market with inferior product, collapsing world prices.[3]

Coffee is a huge industry—it's the world's second most widely traded commodity after oil—and it provides jobs for millions in some of the world's poorest countries.[4] But under these conditions, many of the farmers just can't hold on. Mechanization has slashed the workforce in Brazil by 90 percent. Those who can't afford machinery go bankrupt.[5] In Colombia, farmers who were growing coffee are moving to coca (cocaine) production because they're not making money on coffee anymore.[6] In Central America, the World Bank estimates that 600,000 coffee workers have recently lost full-time or temporary jobs, prompting a flight of Guatemalans and Hondurans to Mexico and a separate exodus of Mexican farmers into the United States.[7]

Reviving Real Food

Buying directly from the farmer is, as discussed throughout this book, the best way to get high-quality products and support growers who are working sustainably. Unless you live next to Juan Valdez, this might feel like a difficult thing to do with coffee. But there are organizations in place that are cutting out as many middlemen as possible to bring growers closer to their customers and are rewarding farmers who are growing sustainably.

And they are using their model to help not only coffee growers, but tea pickers and other farm workers to get a fair shake in the world trade market. (See the Profile on ForesTrade on page 250 to read more about one such company.) Here's how to help them.

Buy Fair Trade Products

A group of organizations, such as TransFair USA in the United States, are working under the guidelines of the Fair Trade Labelling Organizations International (FLO) to stabilize the market for growers by shortening the distribution chain. You may have seen the "Fair Trade Certified" sticker on coffee in the market or posted at your local beverage bar. But it can be used on many food items. It means that:

- Farmers are paid a "floor" price for their products—coffee beans, tea leaves, even bananas—that covers their cost of production and guarantees them a profit regardless of the world market price.
- Farmers may obtain credit.
- Farmers who desire it are paid, at least partially, in advance.
- Organic production is encouraged and those farmers wishing to adopt organic practices are assisted in converting their operations.

Your cup makes a difference. Hundreds of cups make an even greater impact. Encourage groups to which you belong or your office—any place that keeps a pot on—to buy fair-trade beverages. Equal Exchange has purchasing programs designed for church socials and sells bulk products for gatherings as well. You can order at www.equalexchange.com.

Buy Organic Products

Many of the indigenous farmers in the coffee and tea industry cannot read or write. As a result they are often uninformed about the hazards and correct application of agricultural chemicals. Without this information, a percentage of farmers wind up poisoning themselves and their fields through misuse of the chemicals.

The only way you can be assured that you and the farmers are not being exposed to residues from these chemicals is to buy organic coffee and tea. Organic certification guarantees that these products were grown without pesticides, herbicides, or chemical fertilizers.

Look for Shade-Grown Coffee

Coffee is best grown under the shade of a tree. In direct sunlight it grows too fast, which diminishes the quality of the beans. The shade slows growth and keeps soil moist.[8] Organic coffee is often shade-grown because the birds it attracts greatly reduce the need for topical pesticides. Shade-grown practices are also friendly to the indigenous animal populations that use the trees for habitat.

Consider Estate-Grown

The Kona Coffee Council of Hawaii defines estate-grown as "the product of one farm, unmixed with crops from other farms and processed through to roast under the control of the estate farm."[9] This level of control, like that of a wine maker, is why estate-grown products are often considered the highest quality products available.

Know Your Tea

All tea comes from the same plant, *Camellia sinensis*. It is the oxidization of the leaves after harvest—black tea is oxidized, green tea is not—that separates the two. The numerous types of tea on the market are really just describing their production method or point of origin. Tea called oolong, for example, is a combination of black and green teas. Darjeeling teas can be black, green, or oolong; the name means that they are grown in Darjeeling, India. Herbal teas are not really tea but infusions of flavorful items such as berries, barks, or flowers.

Soft Drinks

Our consumption of soft drinks has skyrocketed to more than 576 twelve-ounce servings per year or 1.6 twelve-ounce cans per day for every man, woman, and child.[10] Beverage companies would call that high consumer demand. But is it really demand or is it just the logical response to the ubiquity and iconization of our nation's most popular drink? Until companies such as Coca-Cola and Pepsi got into the water business, you would be hard-pressed to find anything but fizzy drinks in the nearby vending machine. Large-size beverages are now served up in cups the size of small washing basins. And everywhere you turn, from the billboard to the silver screen, cola logos blaze larger than life. What's at the heart of the cola craze?

INDUSTRIAL AGRICULTURE SNAPSHOT

Soda is sweet, there's no denying that. But you might be surprised how sweet. The typical twelve-ounce can of soda contains the equivalent of a whopping ten teaspoons of sugar.[11] Can you imagine spooning that into your morning coffee or tea? It seems almost inedible. The high sugar content has led the Center for Science in the Public Interest to call soft drinks "liquid candy," and soft drinks are being blamed for the skyrocketing rise in obesity around the country, particularly in children who start the soft drink habit at an increasingly early age.

The source of all of that sugar, high fructose corn syrup (HFCS), has a lot to do with the prevalence of these beverages, which I call "liquid corn," in our society. As mentioned in Aisle 4: Grains, Oils, and Sweeteners, and as Michael Pollan describes in the *New York Times*, we have an abundance of corn that is so great, the only profitable thing to do with it is to process it into added-value products such as the variety of processed foods discussed in Aisle 6: Convenience Foods, and into sweeteners.[12]

HFCS, which comes from corn, is the predominant sweetener of soft drinks.[13] Developed in the 1970s, HFCS is used widely throughout the food industry as a low-cost alternative to traditional sugars—sucrose— which are derived from cane and beet plants. It is the extremely low cost of these sweeteners that allows fast food restaurants to charge only a marginal amount more for a tub of cola than for a small child's size.[14] Americans consumed an extraordinary 62.6 pounds per person of HFCS in 2001.[15] That's more than 4,000 percent increase since its introduction to the market in the 1970s.[16]

Manufacturers claim that there is no nutritional difference between HFCS and traditional sugars.[17] Yet there are members of the medical community who beg to differ. George A. Bray, former director of Louisiana State University's Pennington Biomedical Research Center in Baton Rouge, says that "Fructose is absorbed differently" than other sugars. "It doesn't register in the body metabolically the same way that glucose does."[18] The body's inability to metabolize HFCS has been associated with increased heart disease, bone density loss, and rapid weight gain.[19, 20]

Those who wish to indulge in a soda without the sugar often opt for a diet variety. But these beverages, too, have come under fire for the artificial sweeteners they use in their bubbly concoctions.

This torrent of soda pop has removed the preciousness of a product that was once the domain of the corner soda fountain and used to be a treat, a dessert or snack of sorts that was enjoyed the way one might savor an ice cream cone or candy bar. Today, however, soda is often the beverage of choice at mealtimes and as a thirst quencher during the day.

Are soft drinks that delicious? Some would argue no, but they are that addictive. Not as addictive as the original formulations of Coca-Cola that got their name and the little lift drinkers enjoyed so much from the addition of cocaine to each bottle. But most "secret formulas" still contain a stimulant, caffeine, which keeps us coming back for more. And it's not reserved just for brown colas, but is a component of citrus-flavored drinks as well, and often in higher amounts.

The siren song of endless supply and spiked formulas is amplified by enormous advertising budgets designed to increase demand. The "cola wars," as they are called within the beverage industry, are being waged by the two largest soft drink companies, Coca-Cola and Pepsi, to differentiate their nearly identical products through highly funded marketing plans. Each year, these companies lay out billions of dollars to come up with catchy slogans, Super Bowl commercial breaks, and product placement opportunities in popular movies. Their big spending ingrains their logos into the culture so deeply that we hardly recognize them as brands anymore. We just call a dark, fizzy beverage "a coke."

REVIVING REAL FOOD

Nobody needs that much sugar and no company needs that much swing in the food industry. Here are some ways to work around the cola craze:

It's a Treat

Serve soft drinks as a treat, not at mealtimes.

Make Fruit Sodas at Home

I add a small amount of exotic juices like guava juice to plain seltzer water for a fizzy, unusual drink that tastes good and isn't loaded with sugar and caffeine.

Homemade Ginger Ale

This ginger ale has real bite.

One 2-inch knob fresh ginger, peeled and grated
Juice from ½ lemon
¼ cup honey
Ice
Seltzer

Place 2 cups of water in a medium saucepan and bring to a boil. Remove from the heat and add the ginger. Steep for 10 minutes, then strain into a pitcher. Add the lemon juice and honey and stir to combine. Cool thoroughly. Fill 4 tall glasses with ice. Add ¼ cup ginger syrup to each glass and top with seltzer. Stir and enjoy.

Serves 4

Buy Natural Soft Drinks

Look for natural sodas that don't add caffeine to their formulas.

Buy Small

Buy the size beverage that you will drink, no matter what the price incentive is to "super-size it." Send your message to the beverage industry that food isn't disposable, no matter how cheap it is.

When did we all get so thirsty? On average, Americans consume 2.3 servings of bottled water each day.[21] Whether it is in the gym, at the mall, at the office, or on the trail, there seems to be a bottle of water in every backpack, diaper bag, and briefcase I see, including my own.

And restaurants have caught on to our collective state of parchedness. No matter where I dine, the first question out of the waiter's mouth is invariably related to my tolerance or lack thereof for the local tap. Water seems to be "springing up" everywhere—from the old standards Perrier and Evian to new vitamin waters, even rainwater in a bottle. All of this thirst quenching started to raise some questions for me. Here's what I found out about all of those sports-sized bottles of agua and imported waters that we are knocking back.

INDUSTRIAL AGRICULTURE SNAPSHOT

The appeal of bottled water for many is the assumption that what is in that bottle, behind the label covered with snowcapped mountains and under the "guaranteed freshness" cap, is something pure, pristine. Something better, surely, than that sugary concoction in the next refrigerator case and greatly improved over anything you could find running out of the communal water fountain. But how do you know—behind all of the fancy labeling and ad campaigns—exactly what is in that bottle?

You can't rely on government regulation. The bottled water industry, compared to the nation's tap water system, is relatively unregulated. For example, New York City's tap water was tested 560,000 times in 2002.[22] According to EPA rules, there is a zero tolerance for pathogens such as E. coli or fecal coliform in municipal water systems. And the findings are available to the public. Bottled water, on the other hand, is regulated by the FDA, which does not have even one full-time regulator in charge of the industry.[23] Acceptable levels of pathogenic contamination are issued by the government, but the testing for bottled water is governed largely by the industry itself, which isn't required to publish the results.[24]

Outside of purity issues, there are some sustainability elements involved in the water debate. Environmentally, bottled water has been accused of draining natural aquifers of nonrenewable sources of water. And it doesn't take a large leap of the imagination to envision the pile-up of plastic that results from all of those containers. The World Wildlife Federation estimates that around 1.5 million tons of plastic are used globally each year in water bottles.[25] And shipping that much weight in liquid around costs us all in fuel usage.

When all is said and done, however, that's not to say that bottled water isn't the better choice, at least some of the time. What happens between the municipal water treatment plant and your spigot may offer reason enough to avoid the tap. Municipal pipes—which could be one hundred years old—and the plumbing in your house or apartment building all contribute to the quality of your tap water. If you rely on well water, as many in the nation do, the contaminants that leach into your soil may very well make it into your water glass. And if there is a disaster—flood, earthquake, or intentional contamination—you might be reaching for the jug rather than the faucet.

And then there's the business of your personal preference. Taste, convenience, an alternative to sugary drinks, are all valid reasons to carry some water with you. But when you do grab that H_2O to go, there are a couple things you should know. Here's the short list to enjoying a long, cool drink of water.

REVIVING REAL FOOD

Bottled water is expensive—much more so than even gasoline. So when you plunk down your dollars for a bit of refreshment, your bottler at least owes you an explanation of what you're buying. Co-op America advises consumers "to be wary of words like 'pure,' 'pristine,' 'glacial,' 'premium,' 'natural' or 'healthy.' They're basically meaningless words added to labels to emphasize the alleged purity of bottled water over tap water."[26] In fact an estimated 25 percent or more of bottled water is really just *tap water in a bottle* — sometimes further treated, sometimes not.[27] Here are some common labels you might see in the water section and what they can tell you about the source of your beverage.

Know Your Labels

BOTTLED TAP WATER

Aquafina, from Pepsi, and Dasani, from Coca-Cola, are purified tap water. Bottled tap water does not have to be labeled as such if it is treated—filtered or otherwise purified, for example. Contact the manufacturer if you would like to verify the source of your bottled water.

"FROM A MUNICIPAL SOURCE" OR "FROM A COMMUNITY WATER SYSTEM"

If you see this on the label, the water was derived from tap water.

ARTESIAN WELL WATER

Water from a well whose source is a confined aquifer—layers of porous rock, sand, and earth that contain water—which is under pressure from surrounding upper layers of rock or clay.

MINERAL WATER

Water from an underground source that contains at least 250 parts per million total dissolved solids. Minerals and trace elements must come from the source of the underground water. They cannot be added later.

SPRING WATER

Derived from an underground formation from which water flows naturally to the earth's surface. Spring water must be collected only at the spring or through a borehole tapping the underground formation feeding the spring.

WELL WATER

Water from a hole bored or drilled into the ground, which taps into an unenclosed aquifer.[28]

DISTILLED

In this process, water is turned into a vapor. Since minerals are too heavy to vaporize, they are left behind. The vapors are condensed into water again and bottled.

PURIFIED WATER

Water that has been distilled, finely filtered, or treated with reverse osmosis or ozonation to remove microbes or minerals.

SELTZER WATER, SODA WATER, TONIC WATER, OR CLUB SODA

These are not included as bottled water under the FDA's regulations, because these beverages have historically been considered soft drinks.

Install a Water Purifier

Save dollars, eliminate plastic waste, and use local water by buying a water purifier. There is a wide range of purifiers to choose from, from those that attach to the sink to pitcher models that turn ordinary tap water into a better-tasting alternative. There are even heavy-duty, under-the-sink models that promise to render water nearly pristine. If you are interested in breaking the bottle habit, one of these systems might be for you.

Rent or Buy a Cooler

Water delivery services reuse the large five-gallon jugs in which they deliver your water over and over again. If you're using a service rather than cracking open an individual serving bottle, you're cutting down on plastic use.

Reuse

Buy a reusable sport bottle and fill up from your home or office cooler to eliminate plastic waste.

Refill

Refill your individual water bottle from a cooler or tap at least every other time it's empty and you can cut down on plastic usage by half.

Juice

From emerald green shots of wheatgrass to sippy cups full of apple extract, juice is often the choice of thirsty folks seeking a healthy beverage. I'm not equipped to address the nutritional value of these products, but I do become suspicious when I see droves of any new product in the marketplace. Take orange juice, for instance. Juice was juice, then there was the kind with some pulp, and then the type with lots of pulp. Then came orange juice with calcium, juice with extra vitamins C and E and zinc. Now there's even low-acid orange juice for people who can't drink juice. After a point, I start to think that the juice companies are just trying to expand their shelf space in the juice department, not really offer us drinks that we want or need.

There seem to be two opposing camps regarding fruit juices. I have friends who swear by their juice fasts. They start the day with breakfast in a glass and consider a smoothie a good meal option. And then there's the camp of environmentalists, like Joan Dye Gussow, who see a daily glass of juice as an extravagance that costs us more in fuel than it gives us nutritionally.[29] And there are teams of nutritionists who see the overconsumption of juice by toddlers as a leading cause of obesity.

Me? I'm down the middle of the road on this one. I like my juice in the morning but a small-sized portion in those little juice glasses your granny used to have. I give my daughter juice but dilute it heavily or use it, mixed with seltzer, as an alternative to soft drinks.

Wherever you net out on the juice debate, you should know what's in your glass. There is a lot of confusing language in this aisle that could trick you into paying a lot of money for sugar and water, and if you wanted that, you'd buy soda. Here's the juice on juice.

INDUSTRIAL AGRICULTURE SNAPSHOT

Juice is a processed food product. As such, it is vulnerable to the same shortcomings that we find in other manufactured foods. Inferior ingredients, fillers, preservatives, and additives often make their way into these beverages that are widely considered wholesome. Despite the imagery of citrus advertising, it is not the most beautiful specimens that get crushed into juice—it is often the less desirable, often damaged fruits that are utilized in the juicing process, where their flaws can be hidden.

The juice industry is often less than forthcoming with information on the product you are drinking. Tricky plays of words disguise the identity of pure juices behind masks of confusing language. And exotic juice blends often contain very little of the advertised extract diluted in a base of inexpensive filler juices such as apple and grape. Sweeteners are a common addition to juice blends, used to mask their flavor shortcomings. When selecting a juice beverage, it's important to read the label carefully to make sure that you are getting a quality product.

REVIVING REAL FOOD

Buy Local

If you live near an orchard or a grove, chances are you can procure some superior sips. Farms such as these often squeeze their least lovely—but just as delicious—fruits to make tasty juice. Or scour your local farmers' market for a jug to take home.

Be aware that such juice may be unpasteurized—just as it came from the fruit—squeezed and bottled and not sterilized in any way. Although unpasteurized juice must bear the following label: "This product has not been pasteurized and therefore may contain harmful bacteria that can cause serious illness in children, the elderly, and persons with weakened immune systems," such juice is not "dirty." You just have to be mindful of keeping it under refrigeration and know that it will not have the extended shelf life of the pasteurized juices that you buy in the market. Drink it within three to five days.

Buy Organic

Because fruit trees can't be rotated like other crops, and because of the sweetness of the fruit, they are highly susceptible to pest infestations that settle in over the seasons. When possible, opt for organic juice to avoid pesticide residues.

Use Juice as a Flavoring

Dilute juice by at least 50 percent or add just a splash to seltzer to get that fresh flavor while reducing imported concentrates and the sugar/calorie load.

Eat the Fruit or Squeeze Your Own

Get all of the benefits and flavor of the fruit without any preservatives or added sugars.

Avoid Anything but 100% [Fruit Name] Juice

Otherwise you are just paying for sweeteners, water, and inferior juices.

Know Your Labels

Here are some of the labels that you might see in the juice aisle that can be misleading.

100% [FRUIT NAME] JUICE

A quick switch of language can mean the difference between getting a lot of a desired ingredient or just a small percentage. A description that is listed this way—the percentage, then the name of the fruit—is the only way to know exactly what percentage of juice is in the container. Only juice that describes itself as "100% Cranberry," for instance, is all cranberry juice.

100% JUICE

If the label is reversed to read "Cranberry, 100% juice," it contains all juice but not necessarily all cranberry juice; it might be a blend of fruit juices. For example, Apple and Eve Naturally Cranberry 100% Juice is only 15 to 20 percent cranberry juice; the rest of the beverage is a combination of other fruit juices.[30]

BLEND, DRINK, COCKTAIL, PUNCH

Juices labeled with these monikers contain a blend of juices and usually a lot of water and sweeteners as well. Scan the ingredients list for items such as high fructose corn syrup.

FROM CONCENTRATE

This refers to juice manufactured as a frozen concentrate, then reconstituted and pasteurized before packaging.

FROZEN CONCENTRATE

This juice has been concentrated and frozen. It is reconstituted by adding back the amount of water originally removed.

NOT FROM CONCENTRATE

This juice is flash-heated to pasteurize it immediately after the fruit is squeezed. It has never been concentrated.

ALL NATURAL

The word "natural" might lead you to believe that the juice is as it naturally came from the fruit, but that's not the case. Sugar is a natural product and can play a significant role in such beverages.

PROFILE: KANALANI OHANA FARM

Stunning ocean views, towering trees, the gorgeous smells of flowers and tropical fruit wafting through the air on a gentle breeze. Sounds like an ad for a paradise vacation, right? To Melanie and Colehour Bondera and their two small children, it's home. They live and work on a five-acre "agro-jungle" on the Kona side of the island of Hawaii, called Kanalani Ohana Farm. Kanalani means abundance in Hawaiian, and Ohana means family. On their Web site, www.kanalanifarm.org, they say, "We believe that food belongs to everyone and that there should be access for wonderfully delicious, nutritious, organic food for all." To them it's not just a philosophy; it's a way of farming and doing business.

On the farm, their primary cash crop is Kona coffee, which connoisseurs consider some of the finest. Kona, as it is known, is grown on farms like the Bonderas', on the volcanic slopes of the region, and is sold all over the world to people who want an amazing cup of java. Kona coffee is complex and rich, with a slightly spicy flavor. The rocky volcanic land may seem less than ideal for farming, but in the hundreds of years since the Japanese first introduced coffee to the region, it has thrived. The area enjoys bright morning sun and afternoon rain showers year round, perfect for coffee farming.

It has also proven to be a wonderful home to the Bonderas, who first saw the property on vacation in 2000. They'd been looking for a place for a while, having figured out after many years of studying international agriculture and sustainability in the United States and Latin America that what they really wanted was to work and raise their children on a small organic farm of their own. "We talked to a real estate agent who said, 'I have a five-acre, off-the-grid, certified organic farm,' and we thought, 'Well, that sounds perfect,'" explains Melanie. "And within five minutes of physically being on the land both my husband, Colehour, and I felt home. I stepped on this big, huge lava rock, which is the front doorstep, and when I put my foot on it, I had that reverberating feeling of 'I've stepped on this rock thousands of times.'" They moved to the farm in July of 2001.

The coffee, as delicious as it is, is only one part of what the Bonderas are trying to do with their farm. Their interest in international small-scale, sustainable farms fuels the idea of creating a model farm that also serves as a center for people to come and speak about sustainable living. Another goal is to feed their own family almost entirely from what they grow, and although they're not quite there yet, it's something Melanie and Colehour work toward in everything they do. About two hundred years ago, the Japanese divided up the land into five- and ten-acre parcels, small enough for one family to manage, and this tradition has lasted ever since. The farmers in the region, like the Bonderas, strive to keep their land productive and their family lifestyle peaceful and community centered, an important bonus to Melanie and Colehour.

The farm is also home to a coffee CSA, where members pay an annual sum and receive monthly shipments of coffee (a program Melanie hopes will serve as an educational tool to get people interested in a longer-term goal of hers, a traditional vegetable CSA), and an organic apprentice program. One or two workers will come to learn from the Bonderas and receive room and board—not to mention the opportunity to live in such a spectacular setting.

The Bonderas also joined with a group of twenty families in their area to create a "Food Share." Every two weeks, "We go down to the beach and everyone brings a giant basket of something extra from their farm. It could be kale or salad greens or eggplant or tropical fruit. We put it all on one picnic table like a mini farmers' market, and then everyone puts a potluck item on another table. Then we just have a great dinner. The kids run around on the beach, and then everyone takes a bag and takes whatever they want off of the table to eat through the next two weeks at home." The group, aside from being a lot of fun, "has actually been significantly impacting the food intake and budgets of these young families," says Melanie.

Melanie also works as a self-described "anti-GMO activist," working with groups throughout Hawaii on biotechnology issues related to both coffee and other crops. One GMO product being developed is a decaffeinated coffee bean. "The studies show that if you put one test site in this area you could move the pollen out and contaminate the whole region. Kona is two miles wide, twenty miles long—it's tiny. One little test, and we could have decaf Kona forever."

The tropical oasis of Kanalani Ohana Farm may seem very far away if you live in a big city or the suburbs. The idea of pulling a ripe avocado off a tree in your front yard for lunch may seem to have little to do with finding a parking space at the A&P. It may not be possible to grow almost 90 percent of your family's food, as they try to, but Melanie says, "You could literally have window boxes in New York City and grow enough food to have a Food Share with other families. There are lots of ways of doing this." They tread lightly on the earth, respecting it and working with it to reap delicious rewards, for their own family and for people throughout the world who look to them as a model for sustainable living, small-scale family farming, and the production of delicious, abundant food.

KANALANI OHANA FARM
P.O. Box 861
Honaunau, Hawaii 96726
Phone: 808-328-0296
www.kanalanifarm.org

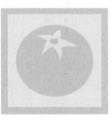

BUILDING A BETTER GROCERY STORE

Food shopping is something that we do most every day, and it can be the single most effective tool for transforming not only what is on our plates, but the landscape outside our windows, the balance of power in our society, and the defining principles of our culture. It sounds like a pretty tall order for what many consider a chore to be crossed off the list after dropping off the dry cleaning and wrangling dust bunnies. But food shopping is not nearly so mundane. As Peter Hoffman of Savoy restaurant in New York City puts it, "Your most important role as a home cook is as an epicure. Procurement is where it starts."[1] And I would add that not only is *what* you buy significant, but *where* you buy it is paramount.

INDUSTRIAL AGRICULTURE SNAPSHOT

The current system of retail food sales in the United States, which is tending toward mammoth-size MegaMarts, supports a system of consolidation that is nudging the small producer out of the food business and diminishing the quality of the food we eat. The entry of institutions such as Wal-Mart into the grocery arena is a major impetus for this trend. According to Phil Howard, Postdoctoral Researcher, Center for Agroecology and Sustainable Food Systems–UC Santa Cruz, "Before Wal-Mart became a major player in food sales the top five retail chains in the U.S. controlled less than a quarter of the market [1997 data]. Current estimates suggest that the top five now share more than half the market."[2]

The consolidation of retail distribution can be traced back as the cause of many of the evils of industrial agriculture discussed throughout this book—monoculture farming, depletion of our natural resources, lack of biodiversity, and an across-the-board reduction in the flavor of our food. That's because huge MegaMarts only want to deal with the gigantic factory farms that share their gargantuan dimensions. As Tom Pavich, a longtime farmer in the San Joaquin Valley, puts it, "[The large retailers] want to link up and buy from a producer that's their size. It's inconvenient for them to buy from twenty or thirty or forty producers." If they do buy from a smaller sized farm, such a goliath often determines the types of crops grown, the harvest schedule, and even the price—choices that are all based on moving volumes of food no matter the quality.

It's standard practice for MegaMarts to charge producers "slotting fees"—remuneration of tens of thousands of dollars—to secure a spot on their markets' shelves. Such barriers to entry in the retail landscape guarantee that eaters only have access to the product lines of the "big food" companies that can afford to pay such fees. As stores such as Wal-Mart push small, local groceries and even midsized chains out of business, producers lose distribution and regional foods disappear from our national food supply.

REVIVING REAL FOOD

While buying directly from the farmer is the best remedy for turning our current grocery model around, it isn't always possible or practical. When your calendar isn't synching up with the open hours of your local farmers' market or you just need a more one-stop solution, the next best thing is to find a trusted third-party retailer that shares your philosophy about food and isn't afraid to color outside the lines of the retail grocery structure to serve your needs.

At these Better Grocery Stores, which include independently owned groceries, cooperatives, and some of the national or natural chains, quality and customer service are top priority. You are more likely to find such items as local, seasonal produce, grass-fed meats, an abundance of organic items or snacks, and sodas that are free of partially hydrogenated oils and/or high fructose corn syrup in these venues. When I'm buying my groceries, I have questions, and nothing makes me lose confidence in my food source faster than an indifferent shrug of the shoulders. At these stores I can get answers. They know if the corn is local, when the wild salmon is coming, if the steak is from a steer that was fed organic grain. They know what quinoa is, on which shelf it is stocked, and can give me a quick recipe for it. Try that at the MegaMart. Many of these better groceries self-publish some sort of newsletter, a communication tool that keeps members informed of its activities, advertises local businesses, and educates consumers about seasonal offerings and events.

Alex Stewart, general manager of Walter Stewart's Market, a family-owned and -operated grocery in New Canaan, Connecticut, summed it up this way, "[Shoppers] want people to know what they like, they want to be treated fairly, they want to find good quality products, they want to trust where they're shopping. And that's what we try to do." Here are some shopping venues that strive to meet that promise.

Support an Independently Owned Grocery

These stores operate outside of the traditional distribution model that you would find in a MegaMart and that gives them autonomy and provides you with better product. Because each store is an independent buyer that doesn't rely on a central buying structure, they have complete control over the items that they carry. And they often supplement at least some, if not all, of their inventory with locally produced items. For family farmers, particularly those who can't or choose not to sell directly to eaters, such models offer a viable distribution solution for their products. As Paul Ryan, produce manager of Walter Stewart's Market, says, "If a farmer knocks at the back door, I can buy whatever he has. [The MegaMart] can't." Paul works with thirty to forty individual vendors for his department alone, visiting producers and cultivating relationships that he's had for years to bring his customers superior products. The meat, dairy, and fish departments all do the same to bring their customers the best quality available. Prized items such as local berries, pies, and cider made from local apples are treasures that I seek at such markets.

Many independent stores are family-owned and as such are inclined to support other family businesses such as the local farm or bread baker. As Alex Stewart says, "We're a family store, we just like to work with people who have hands-on control over what they're doing and are about a quality product." Such relationships bring eaters delicious, carefully produced food and keep your grocery dollars within the community.

In these stores, size *is* everything. It is their smallness—their independence from a corporate structure—that keeps independent stores nimble and able to respond to the needs and wants of their customers. They will often custom-order products on request. It's part of the kind of personal service they take pride in providing. And, as Alex Stewart says, "Because [the department manager] doesn't have to go through ten different layers of management and all the different channels that a large store has to go through, we are able to [respond to customer requests] a little quicker."

Admittedly, independent groceries can be a bit more expensive than the MegaMart. It's the one area in which their size works against them. They just don't have the economy of scale that allows them to purchase tasteless, out-of-season melons by the pallet-load at bargain prices. That privilege is reserved for the MegaMart.

HOW TO DO IT

To find a privately owned store, check the Internet, the listings of your local yellow pages, or your local chamber of commerce. If you're looking for physical clues, privately owned stores are generally smaller than national chains and they often lack the glossy advertising, marketing banners, and "collateral materials" that scream at you in a big store. The only real way to tell, however, is to ask customer service who owns the store, who the parent company is. If they say, "Us," you've hit pay dirt.

Check Out Your Local Health Food Store

Health food stores have come a long way from the days when customers would duck into a dingy scene boasting little more than a haphazard collection of dried fruits, vitamins, and hard-as-rock wheat bread on a few shelves. While it's still possible to find some of those relics from the '70s, today's local health food stores display all the spit and polish necessary to compete against the larger natural food chains.

In many ways, today's health food stores provide the same convenience of bigger stores that sell everything from paper towels to prunes. Many health food stores have a cleansers and paper products section, offering earth-friendly alternatives like paper napkins made from recycled material and chemical-free cleaning sprays.

ORGANIC IS THE MAJORITY

Unlike some of the bigger, more conventional grocery stores where you might have to scrounge for organic alternatives, finally locating some scrawny-looking potatoes in produce, the majority of the produce sold in health food stores will be organic, and say so, and some stores are also starting to promote and label food that is grown locally.

AVAILABILITY OF HARD-TO-FIND PRODUCTS

Many products that you can't find elsewhere, particularly at your larger grocery stores, such as the ancient grains discussed in Aisle 4: Grains,

Oils, and Sweeteners, can be found at your health food store. And if they can't, chances are the managers there will know how to track them down. Health food stores are also great sources for bulk food—a good way of making your shopping experience there more affordable.

DELICIOUS PREPARED FOODS

Many health food stores serve delicious take-away food, a great alternative to the drive-thru, with all the same convenience and more flavor; plus they're local businesses, so the dollars I spend there are staying in the community.

BARGAIN HUNT

Take advantage of sales. The prices at health food stores can be quite high, but the sales prices you find can be just as low. Most stores have a stack of fliers with the day's specials at the front door.

GET YOUR HEALTH ADVICE FROM HEALTH PROFESSIONALS

Some health food stores have taken a lot of flack in recent years for offering unfounded, and in some cases, simply bad, advice about the health supplements and vitamins they sell. As with any shopping experience, it's best to make your purchasing decisions based on the advice of experts, not just anyone.

Join a Co-op

The modern-day concept of a cooperative is often credited to the Rochdale Equitable Pioneers Society, which opened the doors of a food cooperative in England in 1844. The democratic principles of the co-op gained popularity in the United States in the 1960s, fueled by the counterculture movement. Because of these hippie roots, often the term "food co-op" conjures up images of stores that offer only tofu and wheatgrass. But the co-op is neither a relic of ancient times nor the dominion of tie-dye wearers alone.

Co-ops are for anyone who wants more control over the type and quality of the food that they buy. Each co-op is designed to meet the specific needs of its members, so different co-ops can vary greatly. Some co-ops are vegetarian, others sell meat. Some get their products mainly through distributors, others buy directly from local farmers and producers. Some are strictly organic, others sell conventional products. For some, shared work is required, for others it's voluntary. The rules are fluid and open to change as the needs of the group evolve. But according to The International Co-operative Alliance (www.coop.org) a co-op should operate under seven established principles:

AUTONOMY

A food cooperative is an independently run enterprise; it is not part of a national chain, it answers to no parent company or stockholdership other than that of its member base. Whatever money gets spent at the co-op stays in the co-op. It doesn't get siphoned away to fund huge advertising and marketing budgets, pay dividends to stockholders, upsize, downsize, or open an office overseas.

Co-ops elect members or hire a manager to attend to the store's administration and do its bidding in the marketplace. It is this buyer whose job it is to weed through all of the products and claims out there to bring you goods that meet the needs and standards of the co-op at the best price possible. Co-ops, like other independent grocery enterprises, can buy food from whomever they like—they don't have to seek corporate approval or rely on preestablished distribution channels like many national chains. So it's easier for a farmer to get his or her products on the shelf, which benefits the grower and the eater.

DEMOCRACY

Members play at least some role in the decisions that affect the co-op, whether through direct voting with a one member/one vote policy or by electing representatives to boards that act on behalf of the members. Co-ops usually hold some sort of open discussion forum periodically so that all points of view are heard.

OPEN MEMBERSHIP

Membership is voluntary and nondiscriminatory. Co-ops are not just for gourmets or hippie chicks; they're for everybody regardless of race, creed, or social or economic status (or the ability to look good wearing a nose ring).

OWNERSHIP

Members "own" the co-op and participate economically by paying a fee to join and sometimes regular dues to provide the store with necessary operating capital. What would be profit in a conventional store is returned to the co-op members in a variety of forms—discounted prices, maintaining reserves, expansion, or toward other activities that are approved by the co-op board or members. Often co-ops rely on their members to supply at least part of the operating manpower to offset payroll costs. For some co-ops the work requirement is mandatory; for others it is voluntary.

Because the shoppers are the owners, buying food at a co-op can add up to substantial savings in your grocery bill. Co-ops often have a standard markup margin that covers operating expenses but is significantly lower than that of profit-seeking entities. Additionally, the lack of overhead, collective buying power of the group, and often the contribution of working hours by members reduces the price you pay for products.

EDUCATION

Co-ops actively educate their members about the workings of the store through newsletters, meetings, or discussion groups. Free tastings, demonstrations, talks, and lectures are often provided as a source of education to the co-op community.

COOPERATING WITH OTHER COOPERATIVES

One of the guiding principles among cooperatives is the open policy of sharing best practices—strategies for any facet of operation that members have found successful—between stores. By strengthening each outlet, the cooperative model is bolstered. Often managers of an established co-op will volunteer to educate the staff of a fledgling co-op until it gets on its feet.

CONCERN FOR COMMUNITY

You don't even have to walk into a co-op to see that the uniting force of the group is not economic upside alone. Often the windows are so populated with community bulletins that they no longer offer a view. Messages that range from calls to join a political rally to offers of dog-sitting services are all given voice. Members often organize to support local charities and other outreach programs.

The food cooperative is all about empowerment—the collective buying power of a group of eaters to affect the marketplace and fill their pantries with food choices that are in alignment with their personal buying philosophies.

I don't live near a co-op, so I went to pay a visit to Alice Rubin and her place, the Willimantic Food Co-op in Willimantic, Connecticut, to get a taste of the experience. The shelves were a testament to the belief system in residence—a tribute to food produced with care. Organic national brands— Stonyfield Farms, Newman's Own Organics—stood shoulder-to-shoulder with homespun local items like fresh baked breads. Outside, farmers were pulling up to unload fresh-from-the-hen eggs and artisanal cheeses.

HOW TO DO IT

If you are interested in learning more about food co-ops or would like to join one, you can log on to:

THE INTERNATIONAL CO-OPERATIVE ALLIANCE
www.coop.org
The home of the ICA, a base for all co-op activity worldwide.

COOP DIRECTORY SERVICE
www.coopdirectory.org
Provides information about finding and starting a co-op.

Try a National/Natural Chain

Walk into one of the growing number of natural supermarket chains—Whole Foods, Fresh Fields, Wild Oats—and you know these stores are different. The lighting doesn't glare down at you from hundreds of fluorescent bulbs, the decor is appealing, there may even be a local guitarist strumming away in the corner to add to the homespun ambiance. Skeptics say that these bells and whistles are all marketing ploy, a warm, fuzzy veil meant to cloud an eater's critical eye. Even though these stores may not be utopia for those seeking a higher standard in their food choices, the contrast to area MegaMarts is more than just skin deep.

I do a good bit of my grocery shopping, particularly during the winter months when CSAs and my local farmers' markets are on hiatus, at one such store. While I know to keep my eyes peeled—they sell conventional produce as well, and some of the high-end items they offer might not fit too comfortably into my budget—I find it much easier to get my hands on the kind of food I want to fill my cupboards with than I do shopping at the MegaMarts. They have a rotating section of locally grown food that offers seasonal highlights—fresh basil, tomatoes, and zucchini in the summer, pumpkins, apples, and pears in the fall. They don't just carry organic milk; it's organic and local. I can find any number of ingredients—from grains and oils to bread—that are, if not exclusively local, at least from small operations that honor sustainability.

Each department has a sort of "food code of ethics" that it follows; ask your store to share its philosophy with you. In the store near me, produce is dominated by organic selections and everything from apples to zucchini often has point of origin labeling. And while there is still some way to go toward complete sustainability—I don't see a lot of grass-fed meat in the case—the guidelines followed in their meat department, such as no artificial hormones, sub-therapeutic antibiotics, or beak clipping, far exceed the USDA regulations that are standard at the MegaMart.

Higher standards are followed in the processed food aisles as well. You are less likely to encounter additives like artificial sweeteners, colors, and preservatives—there are no nitrates or nitrites in the deli meats. Controversial ingredients, such as partially hydrogenated vegetable oil, have been banned from many stores. Product standards being what they are, the junkiest junk foods never make it to the shelves. That's not to say that my potato chip cravings aren't sated, just that I don't have to read through the labels of MSG-sprinkled, Red #5-dusted crispies to find some salty treats that won't leave me feeling like I signed a deal with the devil to enjoy them.

The product standards cut out a lot of the national brands and that means less advertising screaming for my grocery dollar. Not that promoting a product is bad, but I don't feel like the majority of my food budget is paying for air time. And I'm not bombarded by neon-labeled, cartoon-charactered products blinding me in the aisles—something I particularly appreciate with a toddler in the cart.

Many of these stores have a monthly calendar that is as full as a socialite's in springtime. Educational events—tastings, lectures, demonstrations, and book signings—are scheduled to further the knowledge of customers about their food choices. More esoteric activities such as free shoulder massage, aromatherapy sessions, and talks that address other issues surrounding sustainability such as health and wellness are also offered. Of course there is the previously mentioned guitar strumming on occasion, as well as the random pumpkin painting or apple bob for the kids.

For all the good that comes with this type of store, it is still part of a large company. Not that that is inherently evil, but it does make them a bit less nimble than a smaller operation. They also rely on a good amount of imported items to keep up with consumer demand and to keep their shelves stocked. Read the labels—country of origin tags can be a deciding factor in your purchasing decisions. Imported and specialty items can be pricey. Make sure that you check costs as you go along or you could get a surprise at the cash register. That doesn't mean that you have to drop a lot of cash to shop there, though. In-store fliers often offer great deals. Be flexible in your shopping and take advantage of the sales and seasonal items and you can stretch your dollars.

Create a Private Buying Club

If you don't have one of these Better Groceries near you, you might consider starting your own buying club. I'm not talking about a warehouse like Costco, Sam's Club, or BJ's, but a small group of people who share a similar philosophy about food buying.

A private buying club doesn't have to be a huge, complicated arrangement to bring benefits. A handful of people sharing a bushel of local apples, or a group that orders a shipment of grass-fed meat every so often are great ideas for buying clubs. Those wanting more of a commitment can participate in an established club that orders all of their dry goods on a bimonthly basis or makes weekly trips to the local farm to purchase harvest items by the trunk full.

Groups that already congregate on a regular basis, such as your coworkers, church group, or social club, are ideal for easy distribution, as they don't have to make a special trip for pickup. A neighborhood buying club is also a great option for this reason, but any group of friends or associates will do.

The group will realize substantial savings by consolidating their purchasing power.

Rather than making selections from only those offered at the Mega-Mart, your buying club will be making purchases based on precisely the kind of food in which you are interested, so you have more control over your food decisions. You can also broker deals directly with growers and producers so you will have more access to information about your food and more control over the quality that is acceptable to you.

HOW TO DO IT

Whatever kind of arrangement your club has, a few guidelines should be established so that everyone is clear. These items can be outlined in a simple invitation letter asking members to join or drawn up in an informal contract that members sign when they join the group. In any format, the following should be addressed:

Set Buying Parameters Establish a brief outline of the kinds of foods in which the group is interested. If they will only be buying organic or sustainably produced items, this needs to be detailed. Any specific requirements—that only vegetarian items will be purchased, that any meat bought be grass-fed, that dairy is local—should be listed as well to make sure that everyone is in agreement.

Set a cost limit so that everyone is on board as to how much money will be spent. Make sure everyone knows how that breaks down into the cost of their individual share. You'll also want to determine how everyone will pay—in advance, at pickup, by mailing a check—so everyone knows what to expect.

Establish a Point Person One person should be designated the order collector and placer. Generally this person pays a little less or gets a free share for the amount of work involved in this role. The point person role can be turned over on a regular basis to share the workload and give everyone a chance at the additional price break.

Name a Distributor You can buy in bulk from a number of outlets. Natural food warehouses (see www.coopdirectory.org for a list of distributors) and even some retailers will give you price breaks for placing large orders. But if you are going to be buying fresh items—meat, produce, or dairy—your club would be best served by going directly to the source and buying from the producer. Farmers are often glad to supply a club, as they get the benefit of selling direct and also the reduced paperwork of filling a bulk order rather than many individual requests.

Develop a Distribution Plan When the bulk order arrives, you will need several hands to divide the order and man the distribution point. It's best to have a few volunteers to help out on each occasion rather than trying to organize everyone in the group.

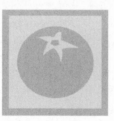

A NOTE ON IMPORTS

Imports are not always bad. But how can that be, considering how hard this book beats the "eat local, eat seasonal" drum? Well, in a number of ways imports can be instrumental in preserving local traditions and communities as well as in filling in some culinary gaps.

Crops such as coffee and tea, for example, can be grown on a small scale and provide a living for local populations. As long as importers aren't exploiting these communities, the import/export relationship can be mutually beneficial. As we discussed in Aisle 7: Beverages, Fair Trade labeling guarantees that, among other beneficial practices, such producers are getting a fair price for their goods. In cases where trade is fair and equitable, the exporter gets to make his living growing a local crop and importers get to enjoy a treat that doesn't grow in their local climate.

Imports can also support individual craftspeople who are keeping an age-old tradition or breed from extinction. The organization Slow Food (www.slowfood.com) scours the globe to locate and preserve dying breeds like the Olympia Native oyster and the Pixie tangerine. Rather than showcasing these products in a museum or archive-type setting, they encourage local producers to adopt them so they can be enjoyed by food enthusiasts for years to come. If the sale of these items was limited to the local communities where they are discovered, they would surely die off—they need the greater attention and care of a wider audience than their existing consumer base can provide.

As the demand for authentically produced food grows, so does the selection of delicious, cared-for items. However, there will always be some products that can only come from one region or from one locally protected process. Certain wines from ancient vineyards, for example, will always be prized. If their producers can make more than their communities can drink, they should have the right to export their product, and those who enjoy such finery should be able to obtain it.

And imports can bring variety to the plate. Spices, in addition to providing a living to a local community and being geographically specific, can transform a diet of local, seasonal selections—no matter how limited—into a culinary odyssey. Take the meager potato, for example. Add a little curry powder and it can be the base for a vegetarian casserole, dice it and then sauté it with some chiles and you have a spicy side dish, roast it in chunks with a sprinkle of oregano and serve it with some eggs for breakfast. And as Joan Dye Gussow points out in her book, *This Organic Life: Confessions of a Suburban Homesteader,* spices are light so they don't require a lot of energy in shipping to get to your kitchen. But even for more fuel-intensive items, such as produce, there are exceptions. I wouldn't want any Yankee to live life without ever having tasted a kiwi—even if that person never makes it to New Zealand.

The trouble with imports is that they are no longer a treat or specialty item. Importing is wrong when it costs local producers their livelihoods. When Hudson Valley farmers can't sell their delicious, fresh, local apples for a profit because area stores opt to stock those imported from China. When we lose track of our seasons—asparagus is not a winter vegetable—

because we are importing the contents of our produce drawer from foreign climes all winter long. This is when importing gets out of hand.

Here's how you can enjoy imported items while still respecting a local food chain.

Support Fair Trade

Look for the Fair Trade label (see below) when you are buying imported items. It's your guarantee that your purchase supports the grower. It is already being used widely on coffee, tea, chocolate, and some fruits such as bananas.

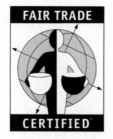

Buy Local Over Imported Whenever There Is a Choice

When faced with the choice of two similar items—the local versus imported, buy the local. As discussed in Aisle 1: The Produce Bins, the local version is bound to be fresher, not having had to withstand the rigors of travel, and you will be supporting area growers.

Savor Imports as Treats, Not Staples

One of my favorite treats is a wedge of fine cheese, with some bread, wine, and good company. Sometimes the cheese—perhaps a French

Epoisses or some Stilton from the United Kingdom—has traveled a distance to get to me. I honor that travel by giving the meal my full attention, savoring every bite and appreciating the food's heritage. But more often than not and for everyday snacking, I rely on one of the selections from nearby Cato Corner Farm—maybe a Vermont cheddar or goat cheese from upstate New York.

Only Support the Best in Class

Save your import dollars for items that are truly tasty. Don't waste your money on Mexican strawberries that are as hard as rocks or year-round tomatoes that taste like cardboard and have the texture of paste. Import only those items that are truly the best, that bring you something that you just can't have locally any time of year, and that are worth the time, effort, and energy spent to carry them across the globe to your table.

PROFILE: FORESTRADE

To many eaters, that sprinkling of cinnamon on their morning cappuccino or those tiny flecks of black pepper on their salad may seem to be just as they appear—small and insignificant. But the fact is, in this country we consume more and more spices every year—close to a billion pounds—and the impact of spice production on the world is tremendous. Spice production, which is origin- and region-specific, mainly takes place outside of the United States—cinnamon in Sumatra, pepper in Malaysia, for example. Many of these spice-growing areas are located in fragile, tropical ecosystems, where the impact from nonorganic and unsustainable agriculture can be devastating to the land, the environment, and the people who live there.

Enter ForesTrade, an innovative company based in Brattleboro, Vermont, where cofounders Thomas Fricke and his wife, Sylvia Blanchet, have reached across international boundaries to create a business model where everybody wins. The company connects some six thousand local, indigenous farmers with international organic markets, providing a high-quality, certified organic product and at the same time, directly supporting sustainable agriculture abroad. They directly source and import organic tropical spices, vanilla, and essential oils, as well as organic and Fair Trade coffee, primarily from Indonesia and Guatemala. Counting among their wholesale U.S. customers are Ben and Jerry's, Peet's Coffee, Golden Temple, and Tazo Tea. They are the largest supplier of organic spices in the United States and Europe and a leading supplier of single origin, Fair Trade coffee.

The linchpin of their success is the fact that ForesTrade combines solid business practices with a social and environmental mission. The company pays farmers a fair price, which exceeds what they would receive elsewhere, and an "organic bonus." These bonuses are used by individual farmers and their producer associations toward a number of improvements both on the farms and in the communities. In return the farmers agree to practice organic, sustainable farming and to honor the national park and rainforest boundaries. ForesTrade provides farmers with the necessary training and technical support to help them transition to and maintain organic farming practices. ForesTrade also facilitates the huge amount of paperwork that must be completed in order for a farm to be certified organic.

"I believe we make a profound and positive impact in the field," says Sylvia. "We know the farmers end up with a greater income while they are supporting the health of their ecosystem." With their increased incomes, she continues, farmers have used the money to "do things like build community centers, create credit unions, renovate roads, establish potable water systems, and renovate community mosques. They've built a lot of mini-processing plants and have been able to buy trucks, so they're not anywhere near as dependent on middlemen. They can keep a lot more of the income in their communities. We've seen the communities just blossom."

And for the eater ForesTrade provides a safe, delicious product. In addition to implementing organic standards, they work to reduce the need for postharvest fumigation or irradiation of the spices by ensuring that the environment at the source is as sanitary as possible, and by taking care after harvest to maintain a high level of quality. Unlike conventional producers who employ potentially environmentally harmful sterilization methods that include treatment with radiation or chemicals such as methyl bromide, ForesTrade relies on natural forms of sterilization, like steam, ozone, and ultraviolet light, which have no negative impact on the environment, leave no residue on the spices, and keep their flavor intact.

The company is applauded around the world for its work. In 2002 the United Nations awarded them the prestigious World Summit Award for Sustainable Development Partnerships. What they really want, however, is the attention and loyalty of eaters. "We could not do what we're doing in the field unless one individual after another decided to pay that little bit more for the organic," says Sylvia. "Every single time it's a choice, and it's such an important choice. People in the United States, when they think of 'organic,' they think 'no pesticides,' they're thinking about their health. These are truly good reasons, but there is always a much bigger picture. I want consumers to realize what a significant impact their buying decisions have on the farming communities in the United States and around the world where organic food is grown. Our products come from fragile, tropical ecosystems. Practicing organic and sustainable agriculture, and paying farmers fair prices for their products, makes an enormous difference to the environment and to the lives of the people who live there."

FORESTRADE, INC.—U.S. OFFICE
41 Spring Tree Road
Brattleboro, Vermont 05301
Phone: 800-989-4399
www.forestrade.com

CONCLUSION:
YOU ARE THE
REAL FOOD REVIVAL

You can eat like a king (or queen)—today. Right now, put down that out-of-season melon, that processed chicken nugget, that fizzy concoction of chemicals. You can fill your plate with Real Food and you don't have to wait for agribusiness to stop growing monocultures, to stop tampering with DNA, or to stop leading government organizations around by the nose to begin enjoying it.

You can start small. The important thing is just that you start. A trip to the fishmonger. A run through the farmers' market. You might get there once a month, or once per season, or you might find that after you eat Real Food, you just can't stomach pale, conventional offerings any longer. A home-cooked, sit-down dinner may not be in the cards for you every night of the week. But a Sunday afternoon ritual of gathering family and friends around the table might just be doable. Don't be afraid to experiment. How many times have you driven past that little butcher shop or walked past the town bakery without stopping in? It only takes one visit to see if their goods might be worth the effort. If you don't like the looks of what's on display, you can always just walk right out, but chances are you will find a level of service and freshness that you thought no longer existed.

Does it take time and money? Yes, it does. But not more than you can afford. There are plenty of meals you can whip up from Real ingredients in less time than it would take for pizza delivery. Scrambling up some farm-fresh eggs is quicker than a run through the drive-thru. Getting a chicken ready to roast—about fifteen minutes. Frying up a steak—no more than half an hour, and that includes time for the meat to rest, a salad to be tossed, and for a jump-start on a good glass of wine. Real Food actually makes food preparation easy—you don't have to do much to quality ingredients to make them taste good.

But quality costs, you might say. That is precisely the point. As the saying goes, "You get what you pay for." Not that your food budget should break the bank—Real Food is not precious or gourmet—but you might find that some items cost a bit more than conventional selections. Try to think of quality rather than quantity. A farmer once commented to me that she has a hard time getting customers to pay a few more pennies per pound for her organic items, but they wouldn't hesitate to drop ten dollars for a fistful of wildflowers on sale at the farmers' market. We need to get our priorities straight. Maybe put down our posies and pay a fair price for Real Food.*

It may take a little effort to gather your provisions, but the more that eaters are dedicated to enjoying Real Food, the easier it will be to come by. In the course of researching this book, I visited a lot of grocery stores. More often than not, the stores that had the largest displays of local food were in regions where farmers' markets and farmstands were plentiful.

---

*For those whose grocery dollars are a little stretched, Real Food can still be within reach. Many farmers' markets take food stamps, many CSA farms have working shares, and many large cities are now sponsoring community gardens that allow residents to farm their own food.

The store managers knew that if they didn't stock bushels of sweet corn, local tomatoes, and the like, their shoppers would have no trouble finding them elsewhere. A steady stream of requests in the suggestion box is also an effective tool for bringing Real Food into the grocery. My area Mega-Mart now carries two kinds of organic milk, a small selection of local, seasonal produce, some handmade cheeses, and even some antibiotic- and artificial hormone–free beef. They don't carry these items because someone in their boardroom dreamt up the idea. They do it because their shoppers want this kind of food and will buy it somewhere else if they can't get it at the MegaMart.

Wherever you shop—at the MegaMart, the farmers' market, or with your town butcher and baker—when you choose Real Food, your actions extend beyond your basket. Real Food is our connection to nature—after all, as farmer, philosopher, and essayist Wendell Berry says, "Eating is an agricultural act." Real Food is culture—a lifeline to our heritage to be passed on to the next generation through the tastes and smells of the kitchen. Real Food is the social glue that binds us together as we gather around the table to eat and drink, talk and laugh. It is our nourishment, our pleasure, and at its best, our passion.

For all of these reasons, we must not relegate the care of our food supply to corporate entities that are motivated more by dollars and cents than our well-being. We must not be complacent in our food choices, because to do so not only relinquishes our power in the marketplace, but in many areas of our lives as well. Every time we choose the local over the imported fruit, we send a message to agribusiness that we value the farmers in our community. Each time we refuse to be seduced by the berries on offer in January we are telling those same corporations that we value quality. When we pass by processed food we show food companies that the nourishing benefits and sensory pleasures of a home-cooked meal cannot be replaced by million-dollar ad campaigns and fancy marketing ploys. Each time we eaters choose Real Food, we *are* the Real Food Revival.

ACKNOWLEDGMENTS

This book would not have been possible without the attention, encouragement, and excellent editing of Ken Siman. We would also like to thank our agent, Lisa Ekus, whose support and incisive advice have been invaluable. And many thanks to those who were so generous with their time: Sylvia Blanchet, Melanie Bondera, David Bull, Lynn Byczynski, Julian Cain, Peggy Clark, Beth Collins, Sue Conley, Ann Cooper, Nicole Cordan, Shari DeJoseph, Liz Dobbs, Sally Eason, Jane Falla, Tom Gardner, Hall Gibson, Walter and Ellen Greist, Richard Haine, Craig Haney, Wayne Hansen, Larry Holcomb, Joe Holtz, Michael Jenkins, Amy Kenyon, Kat Kimball, Nancy Kohlberg, Stephanie Madoff, Tom Pavich, Mary Pat Plottner, Nora Pouillon, Elisabeth Ptak, Claire Rhodes, Alice Rubin, Maury Rubin, Paul Ryan, Tracey Ryder, Paulette Satur, Sara Scherr, Ken and Tori Skovron, Alex Stewart, Lyle Wells, Allen Williams, and Randy Woodard.

—*Sherri and Ann*

I would like to thank my husband, Drew, for your enthusiasm and encouragement, which are manna to me, and for the ride which still takes me further. Thanks to my mom, Nancé

Byczynski, for keeping the faith and my dad, Ray Byczynski. Thanks to Ava and Thayer, my kitchen accomplices. Thank you, Granny Toni, for all of your hours of weeding and tending and for the warm steamy smell of something cooking slow on a cold winter's day. Ann, thank you for giving me the confidence to write this book—your editing brought such focus to the work. Thanks to Michael Pollan for enlightening me and Julia Child for teaching me the kitchen ropes. And thanks to all of the cooks out there, at home and in professional kitchens, who keep the hearth fires burning.

—Sherri

I'd like to thank Fernando and Jack for their love and cheerful tolerance of all my hours at my desk, and for their enthusiasm and support of "Mommy's food book." And many thanks to my whole family, especially my Mom, Alice Clark, for her careful combing of the newspapers for articles relevant to this project, and for her delight in all things delicious, and to my Dad, Bill Clark, who is the only person I know who has made homemade hot dogs, buns, *and* mustard. They both showed me the joy of the kitchen.

—Ann

NOTES

Aisle 1: The Produce Bins

1. In the plots of my community supported agricultural grower (CSA), Mill River Valley Farm, the owner, Walter Greist, still finds shells from past generations of farmers.
2. "Agricultural Sciences," *The Encyclopedia Britannica*, www.britannica.com/eb/article?eu=108625, accessed October 4, 2003.
3. "An Environmental Working Group simulation of thousands of consumers eating high and low pesticide diets shows that people can lower their pesticide exposure by 90 percent by avoiding the top twelve most contaminated fruits and vegetables and eating the least contaminated instead." www.foodnews.org/reportcard.php, accessed May 17, 2004.
4. www.epa.gov/opptintr/pbt/ddt.htm, accessed October 14, 2003.
5. www.epa.gov/opptintr/pbt/aboutpbt.htm, accessed May 17, 2004.
6. "Toxic Herbicide Atrazine Contaminating Water Supplies, While EPA Cuts Special Deal with Manufacturer," Natural Resources Defense Council, www.nrdc.org/health/pesticides/natrazine.asp, accessed November 1, 2003.
7. Terry Devitt Univerist, "Pesticide, Fertilizer Mixes Link to Range of Health Problems," University of Wisconsin-Madison, www.biotech.wisc.edu/education/biotechnews/Pesticide.html, accessed March 15, 1999.
8. Andrew Kimbrell, *Fatal Harvest: The Tragedy of Industrial Agriculture* (Sausalito, CA: Foundation for Deep Ecology, 2002), p. 163.
9. In his book *The Botany of Desire: A Plant's Eye View of the World* (New York: Random House, 2002), Michael Pollan interviews Dan Forsyth, a potato farmer who will not step foot into a field that has been sprayed with Monitor for at least four or five days even to fix a broken irrigation system.

10. Kimbrell, *Fatal Harvest*, p. 71.

11. The Center for Food Safety, www.centerforfoodsafety.org/page302.cfm, accessed November 2004.

12. Brian Halweil, Worldwatch Paper #163: "Home Grown: The Case for Local Food in a Global Market," November 2002, p. 6.

13. As Eric Schlosser reported in *The Atlantic Monthly*, "For more than half a century California has led the nation in agricultural output; it now produces more than half the fruits, nuts, and vegetables consumed in the United States." "In the Strawberry Fields," *The Atlantic Monthly*, November 1995, p. 80.

14. David Karp, "An Orange Whose Season Has Come," *The New York Times*, January 22, 2003, p. F1.

15. Karp, "An Orange," F1.

16. Cornell study, as reported in *Science Daily* Web site, www.sciencedaily.com/releases/2002/04/020412075717.htm, "The longer a tomato remains on the vine, the more lycopene (an antioxidant that inhibits cancer and heart disease) is produced," accessed March 10, 2003.

17. Amanda Hesser, "Salad in Sealed Bags Isn't So Simple, It Seems," *The New York Times*, January 14, 2003, p. A1.

18. Environmental Working Group, "Eat Sustainable, Eat Safe," *Sustainable Cuisine White Papers* (New York: Earthpledge Foundation, Chelsea Green Publishing, 1999), pp. 32–36.

Aisle 2: The Meat Counter

1. Russ Parsons, "A New Blaze of Glory," *Los Angeles Times*, May 21, 2003, p. F1.

2. Matthew Scully, *Dominion: The Power of Man, the Suffering of Animals, and the Call to Mercy* (New York: St. Martin's Press, 2002), pp. 253–255.

3. Michael Pollan, "Power Steer," *The New York Times Magazine*, March 31, 2002, p. 44.

4. Interview with Michael Pollan, "Modern Meat," www.pbs.org, accessed January 14, 2003.

5. Jo Robinson, *Why Grassfed Is Best!* (Vashon, WA: Vashon Island Press, 2000), pp. 8–9.

6. Pollan, "Power Steer," p. 44.

7. Ibid.

8. Ibid.

9. "Backgrounder: Bovine Spongiform Encephalopathy (BSE)," from the U.S. Department of Agriculture and Food and Drug Administration, updated July 10, 2003, www.fsis.usda.gov, accessed July 26, 2003.

10. Robinson, *Why Grassfed Is Best!* p. 26.

11. Eric Schlosser, *Fast Food Nation: The Dark Side of the All-American Meal* (New York: Houghton Mifflin, 2001), p. 198.

12. Interview with Michael Pollan, new content copyright © 2002, www.pbs.org, accessed January 14, 2003.

13. Pollan, "Power Steer," p. 44.

14. Richard Behar and Michael Kramer, "Something Smells Fowl," *Time*, www.time.com, October 17, 1994.

15. EPA Feedlots Point Source Category Study, www.epa.gov/ost/guide/feedlots/, December 31, 1998.

16. Scully, *Dominion*, p. 255.

17. Ibid., p. 276.

18. Ibid., p. 261.

19. Ibid., p. 282.

20. Ibid., p. 249.

21. "Myths vs. Facts About Hog Pollution," www.environmentaldefense.org, accessed February 19, 2003.

22. Jeremy Rifkin, *Beyond Beef: The Rise and Fall of the Cattle Culture* (New York: Putnam Books), pp. 144–145.

23. Scully, *Dominion*, p. 283.

24. Scully, *Dominion*, p. 284.

25. Behar and Kramer, "Something Smells Fowl."

26. Scully, *Dominion*, p. 282.

27. Schlosser, *Fast Food Nation*, p. 196.

28. www.fsis.usda.gov/OA/background/fsisgeneral.htm, accessed May 19, 2003.

29. Elizabeth Becker, "Government in Showdown in Bid to Shut Beef Processor," *The New York Times*, describing the inability of the USDA to shut down Nebraska Beef, Ltd., after it repeatedly failed to pass inspection, January 23, 2003, p. A16.

30. Becker, "Government in Showdown," p. A16.

31. www.ams.usda.gov/howtobuy/meat.htm, accessed May 21, 2003.

32. Joel Salatin, in an interview, www.abcnews.com, April 27, 2003.

33. Pollan, "Power Steer," p. 44.

34. Robinson, *Why Grassfed Is Best!* pp. 11–24.

35. Amanda Hesser, "Challenging Chefs with Odd Cuts," *The New York Times*, January 29, 2003, p. F6.

36. Robinson, *Why Grassfed Is Best!* p. 50.

37. From a phone call to the USDA hotline, April 17, 2003.

38. Ibid.

39. From a letter dated March 8, 1999, and signed by Robert C. Post, Ph.D., Director Labeling and Additives Policy Division, www.fsis.usda.gov/oppde/larc/Organic_Claims.htm, accessed March 19, 2003.

40. www.fsis.usda.gov/oa/background/irrad_final.htm, accessed May 3, 2003.

41. Center for Food Safety, comments to the FDA, posted on www.centerforfoodsafety.org, Feburary 26, 2003.

42. Andrew Kimbrell, *Fatal Harvest: The Tragedy of Industrial Agriculture* (Sausalito, CA: Foundation for Deep Ecology, 2002), p. 53.

43. Sherri Day, "Rip! Zap! Ding! It's a Classic 6-Minute Pot Roast," *The New York Times,* April 19, 2003, p. C1.

44. Ibid.

45. Constance L. Hays, "Here's the Beef. So, Where's the Butcher?" *The New York Times,* February 15, 2003, p. C1.

46. From a phone conversation with customer service, May 25, 2003.

47. Margaret Visser, *Much Depends on Dinner: The Extraordinary History and Mythology, Allure and Obsessions, Perils and Taboos, of an Ordinary Meal* (New York: Grove Press, 1999), p. 153.

48. Behar and Kramer, "Something Smells Fowl."

Aisle 3: The Fishmonger

1. Thomas Hayden, "Fished Out," *U.S. News and World Report,* June 9, 2003, pp. 38–45.

2. Mercedes Lee, Editor, *Seafood Lover's Almanac* (New York: National Audubon Society's Living Oceans Program, 2000), p. 11.

3. From an interview with Mark Kurlansky, author of *Cod, A Biography of the Fish That Changed the World,* accessed at www.habitatmedia.org, June 11, 2003.

4. Lee, *Seafood Lover's Almanac,* p. 11.

5. Ibid.

6. Hayden, "Fished Out," pp. 38–45.

7. www.montereybayaquarium.com, accessed May 19, 2003.

8. www.pewoceanscience.org, accessed May 17, 2004.

9. Regan Morris, Associated Press, www.ocean.org, September 4, 2001, accessed July 13, 2003.

10. David Malakoff, "Death by Suffocation in the Gulf of Mexico," *Science,* volume 281, 1998, pp. 190–192.

11. www.seaweb.org/background/book/algae.html, accessed June 23, 2003.

12. www.seaweb.org/background/book/hell.html, accessed June 23, 2003.

13. Ibid.

14. The EPA bases its advisories on an average mercury level of fish to be between 0.1ppm and 0.15ppm. A Canadian sample of large mouth bass referenced in its June 2001 report, "Mercury Update: Impact on Fish Advisories," had levels of 8.94ppm.

15. Andrew C. Revkin, "Broad Study Finds Lower Level of Old Chemicals, But New Trends Are Called Worrying," *The New York Times*, February 1, 2002, p. A16.

16. Lee, *Seafood Lover's Almanac*, p. 60.

17. www.centerforfoodsafety.org, accessed May 25, 2003.

18. Ibid.

19. Marian Burros, "Issues of Purity and Pollution Leave Farmed Salmon Looking Less Rosy," *The New York Times*, May 28, 2003, p. F1.

20. Lee, *Seafood Lover's Almanac*, p. 57.

21. www.caviaremptor.org/quickfacts.html, accessed June 26, 2003.

22. Francine Stephens, "Seafood Solutions" pamphlet for the Chefs Collaborative, p. 8.

23. Ibid.

24. Ibid.

Aisle 4: Grains, Oils, and Sweeteners

1. www.soystats.com, accessed December 1, 2003.

2. Andrew Kimbrell, *Fatal Harvest: The Tragedy of Industrial Agriculture* (Sausalito, CA: Foundation for Deep Ecology, 2002), p. 142.

3. According to *ABC News*, "Obesity in America: How to Get Fat Without Really Try-ing," December 8, 2003, "Americans consume nearly three times more corn in the form of corn sweeteners than they do in every other form."

4. National Corn Growers Association, "The World of Corn 2004," www.ncga.com/WorldofCorn/main/consumptionData.htm, accessed January 19, 2005.

5. "Agriculture accounts for about two-thirds of all water use worldwide," Sandra Pos-tel, "Dividing the Waters: Food Security, Ecosystem Health, and the New Politics of Scarcity," Worldwatch Paper No. 132, Worldwatch Institute, Washington, D.C., 1996.

6. U.S. Department of the Interior, U.S. Geological Survey, "Land Subsidence from Ground-Water Pumping," www.geochange.er.usgs.gov/sw/changes/anthropogenic /subside/, accessed May 18, 2004.

7. The Environmental Protection Agency has blamed current farming practices for 70 percent of the pollution in the nation's rivers and streams, www.epa.gov/ocir page/hearings/testimony/051398.htm, accessed October 14, 2003.

8. "Twenty-two pesticides have been detected in U.S. wells, and up to eighty are estimated to have the potential for movement to groundwater under favorable conditions," from "Pesticides: Health Effects in Drinking Water," Natural Resources Cornell Cooperative Extension, Nancy M. Trautmann and Keith S. Porter Center for Environmental Research and Robert J. Wagenet Dept. of Agronomy, Cornell University, 1998, www.pmep.cce.cornell.edu, accessed January 20, 2005.

9. "Challenge: Ensuring Public Health by Protecting Food and Drinking Water Supplies," www.environmentaldefense.org, accessed October 14, 2003.

10. Janet Raloff, "Spying Genetically Engineered Crops," *Science News*, week of August 30, 2003; vol. 164, no. 9, www.sciencenews.org, accessed January 20, 2005.

11. Northwest Science and Environment Policy Center press release, "Genetically Engineered Crops Now Increasing Pesticide Use in the United States," November 25, 2003.

12. "Under the guise of CropLife America, Monsanto, DuPont, Dow Chemical and a consortium of other biotech multinational corporations shattered spending records in this small agricultural county. But CropLife America was no match for thousands of Mendocino County farmers, business owners, vintners and families who joined the largest, most successful grass roots campaign the county has ever seen to fight the encroachment of genetically altered crops." Press release, www.gmofreemendo.com/press_releases/2004-03-03.html, accessed January 13, 2005.

13. Kimbrell, *Fatal Harvest*, p. 209.

14. Wayne Wenzel, "Seed Money," *Farm Industry News*, www.farmindustrynews.com/news/farming_seed_money/index.html, accessed November 19, 2003. Details the financing options available to farmers through the seed companies Monsanto, Syngenta, and DuPont.

15. Vandana Shiva, *Stolen Harvest: The Hijacking of the Global Food Supply* (Cambridge, MA: South End Press, 2000), p. 7.

16. Michael Pollan, "Power Steer," *The New York Times Magazine*, March 31, 2002, p. 44. ". . . thanks to federal subsidies and ever-growing surpluses, the price of corn (@2.25 a bushel) is 50 cents less than the cost of growing it."

17. http://ewg.org/farm/findings.php, accessed December 1, 2003.

18. "About $32 billion were paid out by the government in 2000 of which about $30 billion encouraged production and only $2 billion served as incentives for environmental stewardship." Union for Concerned Scientists, www.ucsusa.org/food_and_environment/sustainable_agriculture/page.cfm?pageID=352, accessed October 28, 2003.

19. Abby Goodnough, "Letter from the Everglades: On a Silent Landscape, an Environmental War Endures," *The New York Times*, November 4, 2003, p. A14.

20. *ABC News,* "Obesity in America."

21. Andrés Martinez, "Harvesting Poverty: The Fabric of Lubbock's Life," *The New York Times,* October 19, 2003, p. A10.

22. www.ewg.org/farm/findings.php, accessed December 1, 2003.

23. Andrés Martinez, "Harvesting Poverty: The Long Reach of King Cotton," *The New York Times,* August 5, 2003, p. A14.

24. Andrés Martinez, "Showdown in Cancun," *The New York Times,* September 10, 2003, p. A24.

25. Juliana Gruenwald, "It Isn't Rice and It Isn't Always Wild," *The Washington Post,* November 5, 2003, p. F1.

26. www.mcevoyranch.com, accessed March 23, 2004.

27. Kimberly Lord Stewart, "Virtuosity," *Better Nutrition,* February 2003.

28. Diane Peterson, "Cooking with Gass," *The Press Democrat,* March 21, 2001, www.pressdemo.com, accessed January 20, 2005.

Aisle 5: Dairy

1. According to the 1996 Agricultural Resource Service study, "Effect of Forced Molt and Provision of Lactose on the Cecal Environment and Salmonella Enteritidis Colonization in Leghorn Hens," "The forced molted hens are highly susceptible to Salmonella infection, which results in the contamination of their eggs." www.nal.usda.gov/ttic/tektran/data/000006/86/0000068637.html, accessed May 18, 2004.

2. David Barboza, "Monsanto Sues Dairy in Maine Over Label's Remarks on Hormones," *The New York Times,* July 12, 2003, p. C1.

3. Jo Robinson, *Why Grassfed Is Best!* (Vashon, WA: Vashon Island Press, 2000), p. 9.

4. Barboza, "Monsanto Sues Dairy," p. C1.

5. According to the USDA (www.ers.usda.gov/publications/aib777/aib777a.pdf), organic dairy was the most rapidly growing segment, with sales up over 500 percent between 1994 and 1999.

6. Robinson, *Why Grassfed Is Best!* p. 19.

7. "Pasteurized versus Ultra-pasteurized Milk—Why Such Long Sell-by Dates?" Cornell University, College of Agriculture and Life Sciences, Department of Food Science, www.foodscience.cornell.edu, accessed January 20, 2005.

8. Katy McLaughlin, "Got Raw Milk? Not Unless You Own Your Own Cow," *The Wall Street Journal,* September 11, 2003, p. A1.

9. Robinson, *Why Grassfed Is Best!* p. 33.

10. www.cheesesociety.org, accessed March 18, 2004.

Aisle 6: Convenience Foods

1. Kate Murphy, "Look! We Can Drive and Snack at the Same Time," *The New York Times*, November 2, 2003, p. C4.
2. www.ncga.com/education/unit9/u9story.html, accessed February 18, 2004.
3. Michael Pollan, "The Way We Live Now: The (Agri)cultural Contradictions of Obesity," *The New York Times Magazine*, October 12, 2003, p. 41.
4. www.soystats.com, "U.S. Fats and Oils Edible Consumption 2003," accessed November 8, 2004.
5. Marian Burros, "A Suit Seeks to Bar Oreos as a Health Risk," *The New York Times*, May 14, 2003, p. F5.
6. Tommy Thompson, Secretary of Health and Human Services, at a press conference July 9, 2003, HHS Auditorium, Washington, D.C., transcript available at www.hhs.gov/news/speech/2003/030709.html, accessed May 18, 2004.
7. Burros, "A Suit," p. F5.
8. Amanda Hesser, "Test Kitchen: Homemade or Semi? A Bake-Off," *The New York Times*, October 1, 2003, p. F1.
9. Marion Nestle, *Food Politics* (Berkeley, CA: University of California Press, 2002), p. 22.
10. Murphy, "Look! We Can Drive and Snack at the Same Time," p. C4.
11. Ibid.
12. Ibid.
13. Ibid.
14. Unwrapped, Episode CW1C12, "Microwave," TV Food Network, aired March 29, 2004.
15. Andrew Kimbrell, *Fatal Harvest: The Tragedy of Industrial Agriculture* (Sausalito, CA: Foundation for Deep Ecology, 2002), p. 81.
16. www.ucsusa.org/food_and_environment/sustainable_agriculture/page.cfm?pageID=352, accessed October 28, 2003.
17. Michael Pollan, *The Botany of Desire: A Plant's Eye View of the World* (New York: Random House, 2002), p. 227.
18. Ibid., p. 219.
19. Kimbrell, *Fatal Harvest*, p. 209.
20. Unwrapped, Episode CW1C12, "The Freezers at the Red Baron Plant Are Nine Stories High," "Microwave," TV Food Network, aired March 29, 2004.
21. Eric Schlosser, *Fast Food Nation: The Dark Side of the All-American Meal* (New York: Houghton Mifflin, 2001), p. 4.
22. Bowman, et al., "Effects of Fast-Food Consumption on Energy Intake and Diet Quality Among Children in a National Household Survey," *Pediatrics*, 2004; 113: 112–118.

23. Lizette Alvarez, "U.S. Eating Habits, and Europeans, Are Spreading Visibly," *The New York Times*, October 31, 2003, p. A4.

24. Marian Burros, "Eat Your Vegetables? Only at a Few Schools," *The New York Times*, January 13, 2003, p. A1.

25. Ibid.

26. Ibid.

27. Amanda Hesser, "The Family That Eats Together . . . May Not Eat the Same Thing," *The New York Times*, December 17, 2003, p. F1.

Aisle 7: Beverages

1. Rodney North, "Fair Trade for a Fair Cuisine," *Sustainable Cuisine White Papers* (New York: Earthpledge Foundation, Chelsea Green Publishing 1999), p. 37.

2. Dennis O'Brien, "Cup of Research Is Half-full," *Baltimore Sun*, November 3, 2003, p. 12A.

3. Anne Marie Ruff, "Coffee Is Everything," *Saveur*, December 2003, p. 34.

4. Tony Smith, "Difficult Times for Coffee Industry," *The New York Times*, November 25, 2003, p. W1.

5. Ibid.

6. O'Brien, "Cup of Research," p. 12A.

7. Smith, "Difficult Times," p. W1.

8. Ruff, "Coffee Is Everything," p. 32.

9. www.kona-coffee-council.com, accessed May 18, 2004.

10. Michael F. Jacobson, Ph.D., The Center for Science in the Public Interest, "Liquid Candy: How Soft Drinks are Harming Americans' Health," www.cspinet.org/sodapop/liquid_candy.htm, accessed May 14, 2004.

11. Eric Schlosser, *Fast Food Nation: The Dark Side of the All-American Meal* (New York: Houghton Mifflin, 2001), p. 54.

12. Michael Pollan, "The Way We Live Now: The (Agri)cultural Contradictions of Obesity," *The New York Times Magazine*, October 12, 2003, p. 41.

13. National Corn Growers Association FAQ's, www.ncga.com, accessed February 18, 2003.

14. Schlosser, *Fast Food Nation*, p. 54.

15. Sally Squires, "Sweet But Not So Innocent? High-Fructose Corn Syrup May Act More Like Fat Than Sugar in the Body," *The Washington Post*, March 11, 2003, p. HE01.

16. *ABC News*, "Obesity in America: How to Get Fat Without Really Trying," December 8, 2003.

17. From the Corn Refiners Association Web site (www.corn.org), "Once absorbed, the body has no way of knowing whether a molecule of fructose came from sucrose, HFCS, honey or fruit. Since the proportion of glucose and fructose in HFCS and sucrose are similar, these two sweeteners are virtually indistinguishable by the body," Guy H. Johnson, Ph.D., of Johnson Nutrition Solutions, LLC.

18. Squires, "Sweet but Not So Innocent," p. HE01.

19. Ibid.

20. As reported by Phil Lempert on *The Today Show*, NBC, October 13, 2003.

21. International Bottled Water Association, www.bottledwater.org.

22. Brian Howard, "Message in a Bottle: Despite the Hype, Bottled Water Is Neither Cleaner nor Greener Than Tap Water," *E/The Environmental Magazine*, www.emagazine.com, September–October 2003.

23. Ibid.

24. Ibid.

25. Ibid.

26. www.coopamerica.org, accessed Februrary18, 2004.

27. Based on "Bottled Water: Pure Drink or Pure Hype?" a March 1999 report by the Natural Resources Defense Council, www.nrdc.org.

28. www.fda.gov/fdac/features/2002/402_h2o.html, accessed May 18, 2004.

29. Joan Dye Gussow, "Think Globally, Eat Locally," *Mother Earth News*, Issue #190 February/March 2002.

30. Consumer Reports, "Go Ahead Find the Berry," www.consumerreports.com, May 2001.

Building a Better Grocery Store

1. Baum Forum, New York, New York, May 8, 2004.

2. Phil Howard, "Consolidation in Food and Agriculture: Implications for Farmers and Consumers," *CCOF Magazine*, Center for Agroecology and Sustainable Food Systems–UC Santa Cruz, Winter 2003–04, p. 2.

REFERENCES

You may not hear it from the local anchor at six, but news of the Real Food Revival is humming all around us. Writers, publishers, and broadcasters are using their microphones to inform eaters about the perils of industrial agriculture and delight them with stories about the delicious alternatives that await their forks. Michael Pollan's illuminating articles in the *New York Times* and bestselling books such as *Fast Food Nation,* by Eric Schlosser, and *Food Politics,* by Marion Nestle, unveil the impact that the sometimes twisted intentions of big business and politicians have on the food we eat. Cookbooks like Deborah Madison's *Local Flavors* map out some practical kitchen strategies for enjoying your area's harvest. Magazines like *Saveur, Gourmet,* and *Mother Earth News* celebrate food with a sense of place and taste.

And just below the mainstream media is a frequency all its own buzzing with information about the Real Food Revival. To hear it, you just have to put your ear to the ground, or to the underground, you might say. Here, growers and eaters, cooks and purveyors—those who are working for a sustainable food chain—are penning edifying, inspiring writing on all things delicious. Community-based media, such as online Weblogs and chat rooms unite like-minded neighbors who are hundreds of miles apart. Newsletters, both electronic and print, provide an informal forum for the exchange of information and sharing of resources. Many of these publications are free for the asking, supporting themselves with advertising dollars or through donations. For some, there is a small subscription fee to cover the expense of production. But whatever the cost, the wealth of information in these missives is priceless. These postcards from the frontlines of food aren't just spreading the word about sustainable choices, they're strengthening the movement toward a better food future. (See the Profile on Alternative Media on page 280.)

Further Reading

BEYOND BEEF: THE RISE AND FALL OF THE CATTLE CULTURE
Jeremy Rifkin; Plume, 1993

Although published more than ten years ago, Rifkin's call to arms against the way beef is produced still resonates, and is an informative and thought-provoking look at why we eat beef in the first place.

BITTER HARVEST: A CHEF'S PERSPECTIVE ON THE HIDDEN DANGERS IN THE FOODS WE EAT AND WHAT YOU CAN DO ABOUT IT
Ann Cooper with Lisa M. Holmes; Routledge, 2000

A self-described "white-tablecloth chef," Cooper depicts her realization of the importance of eating local, seasonal food. Her perspective on issues such as the loss of biodiversity and how agribusiness controls our food supply is unique and illuminating. (See the Profile on the Ross School on page 207 for more information about Ann Cooper.)

THE BOTANY OF DESIRE: A PLANT'S EYE VIEW OF THE WORLD
Michael Pollan; Random House, 2002

Pollan, a journalist who writes extensively about food production and consumption, here presents a series of essays. They are all beautifully written and teach much about the complex relationship between man, food, and the environment. The book also offers a profound and careful exploration of the issue of GMOs.

COMING HOME TO EAT: THE PLEASURES AND POLITICS OF LOCAL FOODS
Gary Paul Nabhan; W.W. Norton & Company, 2001

Nabhan's book is an interesting case study in eating seasonally and locally. Both philosophical and practical, the book is a good start for anyone interested in "going local."

DOMINION: THE POWER OF MAN, THE SUFFERING OF ANIMALS, AND THE CALL TO MERCY
Matthew Scully; St. Martin's Griffin, 2003

Journalist and former speechwriter for President George W. Bush, Scully here presents a compelling argument for treating animals with dignity and respect. He takes readers on a fascinating and saddening journey through factory farming, whaling, and hunting, exploring the issues surrounding our treatment of animals with sensitivity and depth.

DON'T EAT THIS BOOK
Morgan Spurlock; Putnam, 2005

I loved Morgan Spurlock's movie *Super Size Me*. It not only focused attention on the potential health impacts of eating fast food but also pointed a finger at other industry practices—such as marketing to children—that can have equally deleterious effects. I can't wait to sink my teeth into this much anticipated book.

THE EGG AND I
Betty MacDonald; Perennial, 1987

Written in 1947, this book is a lively romp through the travails of homesteading on a chicken farm in the '30s and '40s. The author's voice is amusing and perceptive, and the book will provide a diverting insight into long-ago farm life, where many of the issues surrounding food production were addressed in a very different way from the agribusiness of today.

FAST FOOD NATION: THE DARK SIDE OF THE ALL-AMERICAN MEAL
Eric Schlosser; Houghton Mifflin, 2001

An exposé of the role of fast food in the American diet, this book revealed to many readers the horrible conditions in the meat industry. Its length of stay on the *New York Times* Bestseller List is testament to the growing interest in the origins of dinner.

FAT LAND: HOW AMERICANS BECAME THE FATTEST PEOPLE IN THE WORLD
Greg Critser; Houghton Mifflin, 2003

This enlightening look at the influence of a high fructose corn syrup–producing food industry and America's epic obesity problem has attracted many readers, and for that reason alone has taken a big step in rectifying the situation, making readers think twice before they down that next cola.

FATAL HARVEST: THE TRAGEDY OF INDUSTRIAL AGRICULTURE
Andrew Kimbrell (Editor); Foundation for Deep Ecology, 2002

This large book (coffee-table size) takes direct aim at the industrial food model and examines the future of food in the twenty-first century with 58 essays and more than 250 photos. Kimbrell has gathered together a group of eloquent contributors—experts in the field—and the result is a highly informative and illuminating text.

FOOD, INC.: MENDEL TO MONSANTO—THE PROMISES AND PERILS OF THE BIOTECH HARVEST
Peter Pringle; Simon and Schuster, 2003

At once absorbing and troubling, this book doesn't shy away from the complicated issue of biotechnology, from its supposed potential to save the starving to its great dangers.

FOOD POLITICS: HOW THE FOOD INDUSTRY INFLUENCES NUTRITION AND HEALTH

Marion Nestle; University of California Press, 2003

Nestle's book explores how the food industry gets us to eat to our detriment, through advertising and lobbying. It's a sound and scary study.

HOPE'S EDGE: THE NEXT DIET FOR A SMALL PLANET

Frances Moore Lappé, Anna Lappé; Tarcher/Penguin, 2003

Thirty years ago, Frances Lappe's *Diet for a Small Planet* (Ballantine Books, 1985) challenged the way the world eats—particularly its appetite for meat. Now she and her daughter have brought readers an update, providing new information for our modern food consumption.

KNOW YOUR FATS: THE COMPLETE PRIMER FOR UNDERSTANDING THE NUTRITION OF FATS, OILS AND CHOLESTEROL

Mary G. Enig; Bethesda Press, 2000

Even if you don't think twice about what you slather on your toast in the morning, most readers will find much to learn from Enig's fascinating insights into many of the misconceptions about the different fats in our diets.

LOCAL FLAVORS: COOKING AND EATING FROM AMERICA'S FARMERS' MARKETS

Deborah Madison; Broadway, 2002

This gorgeous book takes eaters on a seasonal cooking odyssey as the author travels market by market across the country.

LOCAL HARVEST: DELICIOUS WAYS TO SAVE THE PLANET

Kate De Selincourt; Lawrence and Wishart, Ltd, 1997

This book illustrates in great detail what can be gained—both in terms of nutrition and the future of our planet—by eating locally.

MUCH DEPENDS ON DINNER: THE EXTRAORDINARY HISTORY AND MYTHOLOGY, ALLURE AND OBSESSIONS, PERILS AND TABOOS, OF AN ORDINARY MEAL

Margaret Visser; Grove Press, 1999

A sumptuous look at the ingredients that make up an "ordinary" meal, from sources to history.

THE NEWMAN'S OWN ORGANICS GUIDE TO A GOOD LIFE: SIMPLE
MEASURES THAT BENEFIT YOU AND THE PLACE YOU LIVE
Nell Newman, Joseph D'Agnese, Newman's Own Organics, Nell Joseph;
Villard Books, 2003
From the makers of salad dressing and popcorn comes a practical guide to making sustainable choices about many things, from paper towels to breakfast cereal.

NOURISHING TRADITIONS: THE COOKBOOK THAT CHALLENGES
POLITICALLY CORRECT NUTRITION AND THE DIET DICTOCRATS
Sally Fallon and Mary G. Enig, Ph.D.; New Trends Publishing, 1999
If you've been reluctant to give up that cream in your coffee or a rib-eye steak, you'll find this
book very welcome. In addition to being a highly useful cookbook, *Nourishing Traditions*
challenges many of today's popular notions about what food is good for you. The authors
make a strong case for the much-maligned animal fats, and argue against processed foods.

PASTURE PERFECT: THE FAR-REACHING BENEFITS OF CHOOSING MEAT,
EGGS, AND DAIRY PRODUCTS FROM GRASS-FED ANIMALS
Jo Robinson; Vashon Island Press, 2004
Robinson's sequel to *Why Grassfed Is Best!* updates the information that book so eloquently provided. As well as reiterating the many benefits of grass-fed products, *Pasture
Perfect* offers practical advice on how to find, cook, and store them.

SEAFOOD LOVER'S ALMANAC
Mercedes Lee, Suzanne Ludicello, and Carl Safina; Audubon's Living Oceans
Programs, 2000
An invaluable tool for fish lovers everywhere, this book provides detailed information
about how fish were raised, nutrition information, and much more. The book is great,
also, in that it is extremely user friendly.

SHARING THE HARVEST
Elizabeth Henderson, Joan Dye Gussow, and Robyn van En (Introduction);
Chelsea Green Publishing Company, 1999
If you are especially interested in Community Sponsored Agriculture, or establishing a
CSA yourself, this is the book for you. It offers a detailed look at how they work, and the
positive impact they can have on both eaters and the environment.

SILENT SPRING
Rachel Carson; Houghton Mifflin, 2002
First published in 1962, this is the book that woke everybody up to the dangers of DDT
and the impact of pesticides on our food supply and our health. For anyone interested in
food or environmentalism, this is a must-read.

SLOW FOOD: COLLECTED THOUGHTS ON TASTE, TRADITION, AND THE
HONEST PLEASURES OF FOOD
Carlo Petrini (Editor), Benjamin Watson (Editor), Slow Food Movement, Deborah
Madison, Patrick Martins (Introduction); Chelsea Green Publishing Company, 2001
Mentioned throughout this book, the Slow Food movement rejects the rapidly growing
homogeneous nature of the food industry. Joining Slow Food would be a great way to tap
into the Real Food Revival.

STOLEN HARVEST: THE HIJACKING OF THE GLOBAL FOOD SUPPLY
Vandana Shiva; Southend Press, 1999
Well known for her work in environmentalism, Shiva here presents a concise and com-
pelling argument against the long arm of agribusiness today.

SUSTAINABLE CUISINE WHITE PAPERS
Earth Pledge Foundation; Chelsea Green Publishing Company, 1999
This collection of essays is a great primer for anyone interested in the many issues surrounding food production and consumption today. It's also appealing in that it presents
several different views of the same issues.

THIS ORGANIC LIFE: CONFESSIONS OF A SUBURBAN HOMESTEADER
Joan Dye Gussow; Chelsea Green Publishing Company, 2002
Gussow's tale of her attempts to restore an old house and grow an organic garden are illuminating for anyone interested in gardening or simply eating and living more sustainably. Readers get a close and absorbing look at her life and work.

THE UNSETTLING OF AMERICA: CULTURE AND AGRICULTURE
Wendell Berry; University of California Press, 3rd edition, 1996
An ode to the family farm, with powerful observations of its relationship to American
culture, this book is considered to be one of the fundamental texts of the local food
movement.

WHY GRASSFED IS BEST!
Jo Robinson; Vashon Island Press, 2000
This guide to buying grass-fed meats and dairy products is a perfect companion to *The
Real Food Revival* for meat eaters with a conscience.

Online Resources

There are some terrific online resources for finding suppliers that support and promote
delectable, skillfully produced edibles. Some are the work of organizations started by the

farmers and chefs who spend their days working to bring eaters an incredible edible experience. Other sites have been spearheaded by eaters who are either dissatisfied with the direction in which large scale food production is heading, or simply want to celebrate all of the opportunities there are to enjoy a good meal these days.

Following is a list of some of these resources. You can tap into them for information on exciting events, and lectures and tools for finding more sustainably raised food—all of which are great ways to get more involved in the Real Food Revival.

BIONEERS
www.bioneers.org
An educational nonprofit that strengthens and expands networks of practical visionaries working on behalf of the environment and people. They spread solutions-oriented stories—including both ecological models and social strategies—for restoring the Earth. For example, Bioneers connects eaters with Native American farmers who are raising the heirloom corn varieties of their ancestors. The program protects the corn supply, provides an income stream for the farmers, and avails eaters of this delicious product.

CENTER FOR FOOD SAFETY
www.centerforfoodsafety.org
The nation's leading nonprofit membership organization addressing the impact of our current industrial food production system on human health, animal welfare, and the environment. The Center for Food Safety works to change public policy through public education and legal action.

CHEFS COLLABORATIVE
www.chefscollaborative.org
Chefs Collaborative is a national network of more than one thousand members of the food community who promote sustainable cuisine by celebrating the joys of local, seasonal, and artisanal cooking. Users can search a database of member restaurants that create sustainably produced, delicious meals.

COMMUNITY INVOLVED IN SUSTAINING AGRICULTURE
www.buylocalfood.com
CISA is a nonprofit organization that is dedicated to sustaining agriculture in western Massachusetts and promoting the products of small farms. Eaters can participate in their "Be a Local Hero Campaign" by supporting local growers with their grocery dollars, attending events, and donating to the organization.

Consumers Union

www.consumersunion.org/pub/core_food.html

www.eco-labels.org

You may be familiar with Consumers Union through their publication, *Consumer Reports.* The organization reports on issues of concern to consumers, and their three advocacy offices and Consumer Policy Institute address the crucial task of influencing policy that affects consumers, integral to Consumers Union's mission. Their online tool, eco-labels, provides a matrix of food labels that is updated as new ones hit the market.

Eat Well Guide

www.eatwellguide.org

A national search engine to find Real Food near you, developed by GRACE, the Global Resource Action Center for the Environment.

Eat Wild

www.eatwild.com

Features comprehensive, up-to-date, accurate information about grass-fed and organic beef, pork, lamb, bison, dairy products, and poultry. It also features the country's most extensive list of suppliers of pasture-raised products.

Environmental Working Group

www.ewg.org

This group's team of scientists, engineers, policy experts, lawyers, and computer programmers sifts through government data, legal documents, scientific studies, and laboratory tests to expose threats to health and the environment, and to find solutions.

Farm Aid

www.farmaid.org

A collaboration of musicians, including Willie Nelson, John Mellencamp, Neil Young, and Dave Matthews, farmers, and eaters united to support rural communities.

Farm to Table

www.farmtotable.org

A project of Earth Pledge (www.earthpledge.org), which connects New York–area eaters with growers who farm sustainably. Their searchable database allows users to find area producers by specialty.

Food News

www.foodnews.org

A project of the Environmental Working Group, Food News provides information on pesticides in produce and a printable wallet guide to the least and most contaminated fruits and vegetables in the market.

FOOD ROUTES NETWORK

www.foodroutes.org

FRN provides information about eating local foods and tools for leading local eating initiatives in your area. Users can also access the Local Harvest search engine from this site to locate CSAs, farmers' markets, restaurants, and co-ops that offer local items.

GRACE FACTORY FARM PROJECT

www.factoryfarm.org

GRACE, the Global Resource Action Center for the Environment, works to form new links with the research, policy, and grassroots communities to preserve the future of the planet and protect the quality of the environment. This project works to eliminate factory farming in favor of a sustainable food production system.

INSTITUTE FOR AGRICULTURE AND TRADE POLICY

www.iatp.org

The Institute for Agriculture and Trade Policy promotes resilient family farms, rural communities, and ecosystems around the world through research and education, science and technology, and advocacy.

LOCAL HARVEST

www.localharvest.org

An incredibly useful tool for finding local food. This site includes a rich database, searchable by map, city/state, or zip code, of CSAs, markets, restaurants, and co-ops that offer local items. The site also offers farm profiles and lists of books and other Web sites for more information.

THE MEATRIX

www.themeatrix.com

A project from GRACE, this animated short is a concise and enlightening portrayal of the development and impact of the factory farming system.

MONTEREY BAY AQUARIUM

www.montereybayaquarium.com

The aquarium does more than educate visitors about the fish in its tanks. It provides it formation about the living seas and the importance of protecting their creatures. On this site you can learn more about sustaining life in our waters—an issue that is desperately urgent—and download a pocket guide to eating seafood that is caught responsibly.

The National Audubon Society

http://seafood.audubon.org

This section of the National Audubon's Web site is dedicated to sustainable seafood choices. You can find information on the topic as well as a wallet card for sustainable seafood choices.

National Campaign for Sustainable Agriculture

www.sustainableagriculture.net

A source for education and advocacy regarding sustainable agriculture issues.

Natural Resources Defense Council

www.nrdc.org

NRDC is an environmental action organization that uses law, science, and the support of more than one million members and online activists to protect the planet's wildlife and wild places and to ensure a safe and healthy environment for all living things.

Northeast Organic Farmers Association

www.nofa.org

A nonprofit organization of nearly four thousand farmers, gardeners, and eaters working to promote healthy food, organic farming practices, and a cleaner environment. It has chapters in Connecticut, Massachusetts, New Hampshire, New Jersey, New York, Rhode Island, and Vermont.

Oceana

www.oceana.org

Oceana organizes campaigns to protect and restore our oceans. Campaign teams of marine scientists, economists, lawyers, and advocates seek specific policy outcomes to help stop the irreversible collapse of fish stocks, marine mammal populations, and other sea life.

Organic Consumers Association

www.organicconsumers.org

A hub of information and action campaigns for topics concerning food safety, organic agriculture, Fair Trade, and sustainability.

Organic Trade Association

www.ota.com

A trade organization that promotes organic businesses in North America. The Organic and You section of the site provides information about organic issues for eaters and practical tips for reducing chemical residues through one's lifestyle choices.

Pesticide Action Network North America

www.panna.org

Provides information about harmful pesticides and works to replace pesticide use with ecologically sound and socially just alternatives.

Pew Charitable Trusts

www.pewtrusts.com

Provides unbiased scientific research on sustainability issues such as the introduction of Genetically Modified Organisms into our environment and the condition of marine life.

Rodale Institute

www.rodaleinstitute.org

Established in the mid-1940s by J. I. Rodale as a reaction to the growing dependence on chemical applications in agriculture, the Rodale Institute currently conducts research on developing and promoting regenerative farming techniques. Their motto is Healthy Soil=Healthy Food=Healthy People.

Slow Food

www.slowfood.com

Slow Food is an international organization that celebrates local flavors and works to preserve endangered plant and animal species and artisanal processes from disappearing into the abyss of industrialized food production. Slow Food sponsors a range of tastings, lectures, and other events to enjoy the Real Food they are working to support. Log on to their Web site to find a local chapter, called a convivium, near you.

Sustainable Agriculture Research and Education Program

www.sare.org

A project of the USDA to support sustainable agriculture through research and grants. Their site provides information about sustainability and searchable listings for farmers' markets and CSAs.

Union of Concerned Scientists

www.ucsusa.org

Founded in 1969 by the faculty and students of the Massachusetts Institute of Technology (MIT), this group of scientists conducts technical studies on renewable energy options, the impact of global warming, the risks of genetically engineered crops, and other related topics.

UNITED STATES DEPARTMENT OF AGRICULTURE

www.usda.gov

The source for government policy on agriculture issues.

www.ams.usda.gov/nop/indexNet.htm

Here you'll find the complete text of the National Organic Standards.

WORLDWATCH INSTITUTE

www.worldwatch.org

The Worldwatch Institute does research to promote an environmentally sustainable and socially just society. It is a great source of practical and accessible information.

PROFILE: ALTERNATIVE MEDIA

EDIBLE OJAI

Mountain ledges encase the community of Ojai, California, and groves of orange trees surround its center, an eclectic collection of shops and restaurants. Appropriately the setting for the movie *Shangri-La*, Ojai continues to play the role of oasis for many weekending Los Angelenos and also for the farmers who call it home. Civic pride runs high and community identity is fiercely protected—chain establishments such as Starbucks and the Gap are banned from the city limits. Fertile ground for cultivating the seeds of an eating revolution.

Which is just what Tracey Ryder, founder and publisher of *Edible Ojai*, is doing. This printed quarterly newsletter connects eaters to the local abundance of their community. The inspiration for the publication came from a childhood spent growing up with a grandmother who, as Tracey describes, "grew everything herself or had a personal relationship with those from whom she got her food," and Tracey's desire to have that same kind of intimate eating experience again. Articles on farm policy, interviews with local growers, opinion pieces about the state of the agriculture industry, and recipes bring its readers inside the fold of the area's growing and eating traditions and help them reconnect with the origins of their meals.

Edible Ojai has been so popular that it has become a catalyst for other communities concerned with preserving local flavors who have asked Tracey to help them start their own newsletters. To harness the valuable information and foster further connections between eaters and producers, Tracey has started Edible Communities, an online network of the newsletters. You can find a newsletter near you or find out how to start one your-self at ediblecommunities.com.

THE LADYBUG LETTER

Another publication of growing popularity is the *Ladybug Letter,* from Andy Griffin and Julia Wiley of Mariquita Farm in Northern California. This biweekly missive is a com-bination of practical information as well as some of the best food writing around. It con-nects readers with the news of the operation, offering harvest calendars and updates on farm life, and provides recipes for seasonal treats such as green garlic and stinging net-tles. Additionally, Andy includes essays that inspire, entertain, and educate, but are as unassuming as a midmorning kaffeklatsch. A rant on the many names for broccoli raab (a.k.a. rapini, broccoli rape, broccoletti, and so on), a recollection of a moment of cook-ing inspiration, a musing on urban sprawl have all been given voice in the the *Ladybug Letter.* You can read Andy's work for yourself and request your own free subscription at www.ladybugletter.com.

GROWING FOR MARKET (GFM)

Andy doesn't confine his writing to his own newsletter. The first essay of his that I read was in another publication, *Growing for Market.* This monthly newsletter supports farm-ers who sell direct to the consumer—the growers with farmstands and CSAs or the folks you buy from at the farmers' market. Put into print ten years ago by editor and publisher Lynn Byczynski, *GFM* serves as a virtual community where growers can share best prac-tices—designs for a successful hoop house, display ideas, seed saving pointers—and brush up on the latest standards and agricultural legal developments, or enjoy an op-ed piece like Andy's. As the community of market growers expands, *GFM* becomes an in-creasingly popular and valued tool. You can check them out at www.growingformar-ket.com.

INDEX